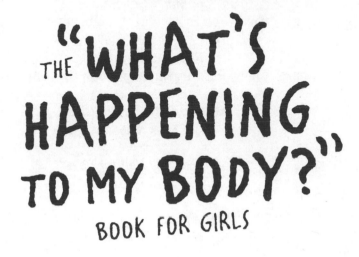

THE "WHAT'S HAPPENING TO MY BODY?"

BOOK FOR GIRLS

OTHER BOOKS BY LYNDA MADARAS

On Your Mark, Get Set, Grow!
A *"WHAT'S HAPPENING TO MY BODY?"* BOOK FOR YOUNGER BOYS

Ready, Set, Grow!
A *"WHAT'S HAPPENING TO MY BODY?"* BOOK FOR YOUNGER GIRLS

My Body, My Self for Girls
AND AREA MADARAS

My Body, My Self for Boys
AND AREA MADARAS

My Feelings, My Self for Girls
AND AREA MADARAS

The "What's Happening to My Body?" Book for Boys
WITH AREA MADARAS

*Lynda Madaras Talks to Teens About AIDS: An Essential Guide
for Parents, Teachers, and Young People*

Womancare: A Gynecological Guide to Your Body
WITH JANE PATTERSON, M.D.

Woman Doctor: The Education of Jane Patterson, M.D.
WITH JANE PATTERSON, M.D.

Great Expectations
WITH LEIGH ADAMS

The Alphabet Connection
WITH PAM PALEWICZ-ROUSSEAU

Child's Play

THE "WHAT'S HAPPENING TO MY BODY?"

BOOK FOR GIRLS

(revised third edition)

LYNDA MADARAS
WITH AREA MADARAS

DRAWINGS BY SIMON SULLIVAN

WILLIAM MORROW
An Imprint of HarperCollinsPublishers

FIRST WILLIAM MORROW PAPERBACK EDITION PUBLISHED 2012.

Library of Congress Cataloging-in-Publication Data

Madaras, Lynda.

The what's happening to my body? book for girls / Lynda Madaras, with Area Madaras ; drawings by Simon Sullivan. — 3rd rev. ed.

    p. cm.

Includes bibliographical references and index.

ISBN 978-1-55704-764-9 (pbk.) — ISBN 978-1-55704-768-7 (hardcover : alk. paper) 1. Teenage girls—Growth—Juvenile literature. 2. Teenage girls—Physiology—Juvenile literature. 3. Puberty—Juvenile literature. 4. Sex instruction for girls—Juvenile literature. I. Madaras, Area. II. Sullivan, Simon, ill. III. Title.

RJ144.M3 2007
613.9'55—dc22

2007009862

Book design by Kris Tobiassen

16 17 18 19 20   RRD   20 19 18 17 16 15 14 13 12 11

CONTENTS

7. ALL ABOUT HAVING PERIODS

LIST OF ILLUSTRATIONS

IN MEMORY OF
YVONNE PINTO,
1968–1999

FOREWORD
by Marcia E. Herman-Giddens, PA, DrPH

Puberty is an exciting but difficult and complex time, not only for the youngsters going through it, but for their parents as well. Lynda Madaras's book *The "What's Happening to My Body?" Book for Girls* presents thorough, open, "child-friendly" information on everything having to do with puberty, from the physical aspects of biological events and how to select the appropriate "menstrual protection" product to social issues such as sexual abuse and anorexia. It not only tells girls what they need to know, but will serve as a communication tool between themselves and their parents. Even though our culture surrounds us with sexual images, even sexualizing young children to sell products, we are still often conflicted and uncomfortable when it comes to discussing puberty and sexuality with our own children, especially now that girls are starting to develop at younger ages than in the past.

Parents will also benefit from reading the book, especially the Introduction, where they will learn ways to discuss puberty with their children. The book is so thorough, many parents will learn much themselves. Girls will especially appreciate the down-to-earth straight talk and the demystification of male and female sexual growth and functions. The questions from real girls in each chapter help make the answers personal for each reader.

This book is especially welcome given the confusing messages about sexuality from our culture and the increased prevalence and danger of the newer sexually transmitted diseases, both occurring at a time when many schools are more resistant to sex education than ever. In addition, access to accurate information is paramount for young people today because social protections that existed for children in the past have largely disappeared.

Instead of the envelope of shame and secrecy that has often accompanied female sexual growth and functions, this book celebrates the attainment of womanhood and promotes the idea of each girl designing a puberty rite to celebrate her entrance into womanhood. Wonderful! I hope this becomes a practice everywhere. Every girl and her parents will benefit from this remarkable book.

MARCIA E. HERMAN-GIDDENS, PA, DrPH
Adjunct Associate Professor of Maternal and Child Health
School of Public Health
University of North Carolina, Chapel Hill

INTRODUCTION FOR PARENTS

My daughter must have been nine or ten when it first started—her introduction to the nasty world of playground politics and the cruel games young girls play with one another. She'd arrive home from school in tears; her former best friend was now someone else's closest ally; she'd been excluded from the upcoming slumber party or was the victim of some other calculated schoolgirl snub. She'd cry her eyes out. I didn't know what to say.

It went on for months and months. And then I finally began to realize that no sooner had she dried her tears than I would hear her on the telephone, maliciously gossiping about some other little girl, a former friend, and cementing a new friendship by plotting to exclude this other girl. I was indignant, and I began to point out the inconsistency in her behavior.

"You don't understand," she'd yell, stomping off to her bedroom and slamming the door.

She was right. I didn't understand. From time to time, I'd talk to the other mothers. It was the same with all of us. Why were our daughters acting like this? None of us had any answers.

"Well, girls will be girls," sighed one mother philosophically. "They all do it and we did the same when we were their age."

The games we played with each other were not very pretty. Exclusion was the basic format. One girl, for the crime of being the smartest, the prettiest, the ugliest, the dumbest, the most sexually developed, or whatever, was designated the victim. She was cast out, ostracized by the group.

On top of this, there was a growing tension between my daughter and me. She was terribly moody, and it seemed as if she was always angry with me. And I was often angry with her. Of course, we'd always quarreled, but now the quarrels were almost constant. All of this bothered me a great deal, but even more disturbing was the change in her attitude about her body. In contrast to the shy wonder that greeted her first pubic hairs, there was now a complete horror at the idea of developing breasts and having her first period. Like most "modern" mothers, I wanted my daughter's transition from childhood to womanhood to be a comfortable, even joyous, time. I had intended to provide her with all the necessary information in a frank, straightforward manner. But here was my daughter telling me she didn't want to grow breasts or have her first period. I asked why, but didn't get much further than "because I donwanna."

Clearly something was amiss. I thought I'd made all the necessary information available in the most thoroughly modern manner, but the anticipated results—a healthy and positive attitude toward her body—had not materialized.

Finally I began to realize that I hadn't given my daughter all the information I thought I had. I hadn't told her very much about menstruation and the changes that would take place in her body over the next few years. She'd seen me in the bathroom changing a tampon, and I'd tossed off a quick explanation of menstrual periods, but I'd never really sat down and discussed the topic with her. I'd read her any number of marvelous children's books that explain conception, birth, and sexuality, but I'd never read her one about menstruation. Obviously, it was time to do that.

Throughout history, in culture after culture, menstruation has been a taboo subject. The taboo has taken many forms: One must not eat the food cooked by a menstruating woman; touch objects she has touched; look into her eyes; have sex with her. We no longer believe in these superstitions, but the menstrual taboo is still alive and well.

Of course, we are no longer banished to menstrual huts each month, as were our ancestral mothers in more primitive societies. But, thanks to centuries of conditioning, we have so completely internalized the menstrual taboo that it's simply not necessary to bother any longer with menstrual huts. We remove any disturbing sight or mention of menstruation through our ladylike avoidance of any public discussion of the topic and our meticulous toilet-paper mummification of our bloodied pads and tampons. So total is our silence that we ourselves are sometimes not aware of it.

During my research into puberty, I have learned quite a bit about the physiological processes of menstruation. But I also learned that I had a whole host of negative attitudes about menstruation, attitudes that had not even been conscious. If I talked to my daughter about menstruation, I could say the right words, but would my body language or my tone of voice betray my intended message?

I worried about all this for entirely too long, until the obvious solution sneaked up on me: I simply explained to my daughter that when I was growing up, people thought of menstruation as something unclean and unmentionable. Now that I was older and more grown up, my attitudes were changing, but some of the feelings I had were old ones that I had lived with for a long time—all my life, in fact—and they were hard to shake off. Sometimes they still got in my way without my even knowing it. This, of course, made perfect sense to my daughter, and from this starting point, we began to learn about our bodies together.

I talked to my daughter about what I had learned about the workings of the menstrual cycle. I showed her some magnificent pictures taken inside a woman's body at the very moment of ovulation as the delicate, fingerlike projections on the end of the Fallopian tubes reached out to grasp the ripe egg.

A friend's mother gave us a wonderful collection of booklets from a menstrual pad manufacturer that dated back over a period of thirty years. We read them together, laughing at the old-fashioned attitudes, attitudes I'd grown up with. I promised my daughter that when she started to menstruate, I would give her the opal ring that I always wore on my left hand, and that she, in turn, could pass it on to her daughter.

One day, as I sat working at my typewriter, I heard my daughter yelling to me from the bathroom, "Hey, Mom, guess what I got twenty-one of?"

We had a pregnant cat at the time, and for a few horrible moments, I was struck numb with the thought of twenty-one kittens. But it wasn't kittens. My daughter was back to counting pubic hairs.

The time that we'd spent learning about menstruation and puberty had paid off. My daughter had regained her sense of excitement about the changes that were taking place in her body. This healthy attitude toward her body alone made our discussions worthwhile, but there were also other changes. First of all, things between the two of us got much better. We were back to our old, easy footing. She didn't magically start cleaning her bedroom or anything like that. We still had our quarrels, but they subsided to a livable level. And when we fought, at least we were fighting about the things we said we were fighting about. The underlying resentment and tension that had been erupting from beneath even our mildest disagreements were gone.

But the most amazing change, perhaps because it was so unexpected, was that my daughter's role in the playground machinations had begun to change. In *My Mother, My Self,* Nancy Friday suggested that the mother's failure to deal with her daughter's dawning sexuality, her silence about menstruation and the changes in the daughter's body, is perceived by the daughter as a rejection of the daughter's feminine and sexual self.

This silent rejection of these essential elements of self, coming as it does just at the time in the daughter's life when these very aspects of femininity and sexuality are manifesting themselves in the physical changes of her body, is nothing short of devastating. The daughter feels an overwhelming sense of rejection from the figure in her life with whom she is most intensely identified. One of the ways in which the daughter seeks to cope, to gain some control over her emotional life, is through the psychodramas of rejection that she continually reenacts with her peers.

I believe my daughter perceived my attention to the changes taking place in her body as an acceptance of her sexual self, and this, in turn, lessened her need to participate in these playground psychodramas of rejection.

I wouldn't want to go so far as to promise you that spending time teaching your daughter about menstruation and the other physical changes of puberty will magically deliver her from the psychodramatics of puberty or will automatically erase the tensions that so often exist between parents and their adolescent daughters. But my experiences with my own daughter—and later as the teacher of classes on puberty and sexuality for teens and preteens—have convinced me that kids of this age need and want lots of information about what is happening to them at this point in their lives.

Beyond providing the basic facts, I hope that this book will help parents and daughters get past the "embarrassment barrier."

Ideally, I imagine parents sitting down and reading it with their daughters. Somehow, having the facts printed on a page makes it less embarrassing—someone else is saying it, not you; you're just reading the information.

Of course, it's not necessary for both parents to read the book with their daughter. Either one parent or the other may choose to do so, or it may work better in your particular situation for you to simply give the book to your daughter to read on her own.

Regardless of whether you read it separately or together, I hope you'll find a way to talk with your daughter about the changes that are—or soon will be—taking place in her body. Kids often have minute and detailed concerns about these changes. Kids of this age need lots of reassurance that what's happening to them is perfectly normal.

It's been my experience that kids are enormously grateful for such reassurance. I actually have had classes where kids burst into spontaneous applause when I walked into the room. I also have file drawers full of touching letters from readers thanking me for having allayed some fear or doubt of theirs.

Not only are kids grateful when their needs for reassurance are met in that way, but they also develop a profound respect for and trust in the source of that reassurance. Parents need to realize what a powerful bond they can forge with their children if they will "be there" for daughters during puberty—not to mention how well the ensuing trust and respect will serve all concerned in later years when your daughter is faced with making decisions about sex. If you're there for your kid when she's wondering, she's more likely to come to you for advice when she's deciding.

Having said all this, I should also warn you that even after your daughter has read the book, talking to her about puberty changes may not be the easiest thing to do. If you come at it head-on by asking a direct question—"What did you think of the book?" or "Is there anything in the book you'd like to talk about?"—it's likely that you'll get something along the lines of, "It was okay," or "Naw, there's nothin' I want to know," or "I donwanna talk about that stuff." In my experience, it's better to take a slightly different approach. Start things off by talking about one of your own puberty experiences. Tell a story about something embarrassing or stupid that happened to you.

By using this approach, you make it easier for your kid to open up. By virtue of whatever embarrassing, dumb story you've told about yourself, you've let her know that it's okay to be uncertain and less than all-knowingly perfect about the whole business.

Here's another pearl of wisdom: Avoid having one all-purpose "talk." It won't fill the bill, no matter how hard you try. It's better to approach things casually, bringing up the topic from time to time when it seems natural to do so. In my experience, a more casual, spur-of-the-moment approach to talking to your child about puberty works better.

Yet another piece of advice: If talking about puberty and sexuality is difficult or embarrassing for you, say so. There's nothing wrong with telling your child, "This is really embarrassing for me," or "My parents never talked to me about this stuff, so I feel kind of weird trying to talk to you," or whatever. Your child is going to pick up on your embarrassment anyway from your tone of voice, your body language, or any one of the other ways we have of communicating what we're really feeling. By trying to pretend you're not uncomfortable, you'll only succeed in confusing your child. Once you've admitted your feelings, you've cleared the air.

As a parent, you may find that you have some concerns about some of the material covered in this book. Some of the topics are very controversial. When controversial questions come up in class, I try to present the various points of view and explain why people have them. I think I do a pretty good job of being objective, but sometimes my own point of view may come through. You may find that your opinion on some of the topics covered in this book is different from mine, but this doesn't mean you have to throw the baby out with the bathwater. Instead, you can use these differences as an opportunity to explain your own attitudes and values to your child.

New research has shown that girls are beginning puberty earlier. As a consequence we want this book to be accessible to younger girls. This is consistent with my overall understanding of the strong need for early puberty education. It is my firm belief that kids who aren't given reassuring puberty education when they need it do not later respond as well to their parents' or schools' efforts to impart moral codes or even just safe, sane guidelines for sexual conduct. In this book we emphasize puberty changes and touch only lightly on traditional "sex education" material.

Regardless of how you decide to deal with the topics of puberty and sexuality or how you decide to use the book, I hope that it will help you and your child gain a greater understanding of the process of puberty and that it will bring the two of you closer together.

1.
PUBERTY

I kept wanting it to happen. When it did I remember thinking, "It's about time." It was late for me and I was really stressed. I was relieved when It finally happened.

—KAREN, AGE 36

Beforehand, I didn't want to at all. I kept hoping I would be the last one.

—SARA, AGE 28

I remember my brothers weren't allowed to hit me in the chest anymore. I was kind of pleased about that.

—JULIE, AGE 53

I was worried at first. Then it really wasn't so bad after all. It just wasn't as big a deal as everyone made out.

—MICHELLE, AGE 23

These women are all talking about the same thing: *puberty*.* Puberty is the time in your life when your body is changing from a child's body into an adult's body.

---

puberty (PEW-bur-tee). You say "puberty" with the most emphasis on the first part of the word, PEW.

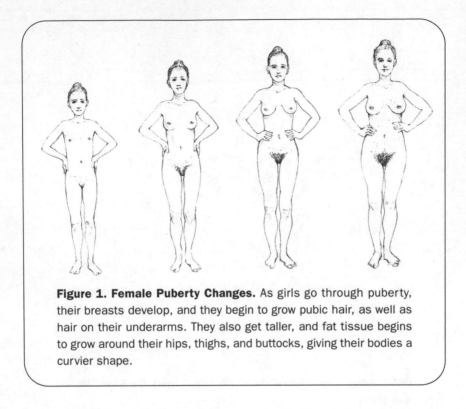

Figure 1. Female Puberty Changes. As girls go through puberty, their breasts develop, and they begin to grow pubic hair, as well as hair on their underarms. They also get taller, and fat tissue begins to grow around their hips, thighs, and buttocks, giving their bodies a curvier shape.

As you can see from Figure 1, our bodies change quite a bit as we go through puberty. We grow taller. Of course, we grow taller all throughout childhood. But, during puberty, a girl goes through a growth spurt. She grows taller, at a faster rate, than she ever will again.

During puberty the shape of our bodies changes. Our breasts begin to swell and to blossom out from our chests. Our

---

There are a number of words in this book that we think you may not have heard before. When we first use these words, you'll find a pronunciation key at the bottom of the page. We will always use capital letters to indicate which part of the word to emphasize when you say it out loud. And we use "uh" in the pronunciation guide to indicate the vowel sound that rhymes with the "uh" in "huh." See, for example, "vulva," "testicles," and "urethra." Remember that you don't pronounce the "h" in "uh."

hips and thighs get wider. We take on a more rounded, curvy shape. Soft nests of hair begin to grow between our legs and under our arms. Our skin begins to make new oils, which change the very feel and smell of us. While these changes are happening on the outside of our bodies, other changes are happening on the inside.

For some girls, puberty seems to take forever. For others, these changes happen so fast they seem to take place overnight. They don't really happen that quickly, though. Puberty happens slowly and gradually, over a period of many months and years. The first changes may start when a girl is quite young, or may not begin until her teen years.

No matter when puberty starts for you, we bet you'll have lots of questions about what's happening to your body. We hope this book will answer those questions.

"We" are my daughter, Area, and I. The two of us worked together to write this book. We talked to doctors and read medical books. And we talked to many women and girls, too. They told us what happened to them during puberty, how they felt, and what questions they had. I teach classes in puberty, and together Area and I do workshops on puberty for kids and their parents. The kids in my classes and the mothers and daughters in our workshops always have lots of questions. They also have lots to say about puberty. Their quotes appear throughout these pages,* so, in a sense, they helped write this book.

I first began teaching puberty and sexuality classes back in the days when dinosaurs still roamed the Earth (well, nearly that long ago). Back then, sex education wasn't taught in very many

---

*To protect their privacy, we changed the names of the girls and women who were kind enough to let us quote them.

schools. I had to invent my lesson plans from scratch. I decided to start off my very first class by explaining how babies are made. This seemed like a good place to begin. After all, during puberty, your body is getting ready for a time in your life when you may decide to have a baby.

I didn't think I'd have any problems teaching that first class. "Nothing to it," I told myself. "I'll just go in there and start by talking to the kids about how babies are made. No problem."

Boy, was I wrong! I'd hardly opened my mouth before the class went crazy. Kids were giggling, nudging each other, and getting red in the face. One boy even fell off his chair.

The class was acting weird because to talk about how babies are made, I had to talk about sex. Sex, as you may have noticed, is a *very big deal*. People often act embarrassed, giggly, or strange when the topic of sex comes up.

SEX

The word *sex* itself is confusing. Even though it's a small word, *sex* has a lot of meanings. In its most basic meaning, *sex* simply refers to the different bodies males and females have. There are lots of differences between male and female bodies. The most obvious is that males have a *penis* and a *scrotum,* and females have a *vulva* and a *vagina.* These body parts, or organs, are called *sex organs.* People have either male or female sex organs and belong to either the male or female sex.

---

penis (PEE-niss)
scrotum (SKROW-tum)
vulva (VUL-vuh)
vagina (vah-JEYE-nuh)

The word *sex* is also used in other ways. We may say that two people are "having sex." This usually means they are having *sexual intercourse*. As we'll explain later in this chapter, sexual intercourse involves the joining together of two people's sex organs. Intercourse between a male and a female is also how babies are made.

We may say that two people are "being sexual with each other." This means they are having sexual intercourse or are holding, touching, or caressing each other's sex organs. We may say that we are "feeling sexual." This means that we are having feelings or thoughts about being sexual with another person.

Our sex organs are private parts of our bodies. We usually keep them covered. We don't talk about them in public very often. Having sexual feelings and being sexual with someone aren't usually classroom topics either.

If I had half a brain in my head, I would have thought about all this before my first class. I would have realized that coming into a classroom and talking about sex, penises, and vaginas was going to cause a *big* commotion. After that first class, I caught on real quick. I decided that, if we were going to get all silly and giggly, we might as well get *really* silly and giggly. Now I start my classes and workshops by passing out copies of the drawings in Figure 2. I also give everyone red- and blue-colored pencils.

Figure 2 shows the sex organs on the outside of the body in a grown man and a grown woman. These sex organs are also called the *genital*, or *reproductive*, organs. We have sex organs on both the inside and outside of our bodies. They change as we go through puberty.

---

sexual intercourse (SEK-shoo-uhl IN-ter-kors)
genital (JEN-uh-tuhl)
reproductive (REE-pruh-DUKT-iv)

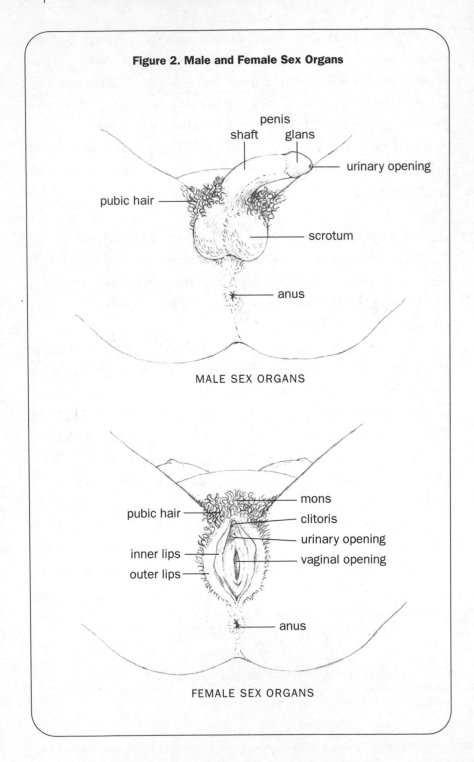

Figure 2. Male and Female Sex Organs

MALE SEX ORGANS

FEMALE SEX ORGANS

THE MALE SEX ORGANS

Once everyone has copies and colored pencils, I hold up the picture of the male sex organs. I tell the class that the sex organs on the outside of a man's body are the penis and the scrotum. The kids in my class still giggle like mad or fall off their chairs in embarrassment, but I don't pay much attention. Using my best Kindergarten Lady voice, I say, "The penis itself has two parts: the shaft and the *glans*. Find the shaft of the penis and color it with blue and red stripes." Now everybody gets very intent on the coloring. Some are still giggling, but they do start coloring. Why don't you color the shaft in, too? (Unless, of course, this book belongs to someone else or to a library. One of the people we most admire is a librarian named Lou Ann Sobieski. We would be in *very hot water* if Lou Ann thought we were telling people to color library books. If this book isn't yours, make a copy of the page to color.)

Next I ask the class to find the small slit at the tip of the penis and circle it in red. This is the *urinary* opening. It is the opening through which *urine* (pee) leaves the body. There's usually less giggling by now. The urinary opening is small. The class has to pay more attention to the coloring.

Then we color in the glans itself. I usually suggest blue, but color it any way you want.

"Red and blue polka dots for the scrotum," I tell my class next. The scrotum is a loose bag of skin that lies beneath the penis. *Scrotal sac* is another name for the scrotum. Inside the scrotum are two egg-shaped organs called *testes*, or *testicles*. (You can't

---

glans (GLANZ)
urinary (YOUR-in-air-ee)
urine (YOUR-in)
scrotal sac (SKROW-tuhl SAK)
testes (TES-teez)
testicles (TES-tuh-kuhls)

see the testicles in Figure 2. I mention them because we will be talking about them in just a few pages.)

Then, I explain that the curly hairs on the sex organs are *pubic* hairs. I have the class color them as well.

Finally, we come to the *anus*. This is the opening through which *feces* (*bowel* movements) leave our bodies. The anus isn't a reproductive organ. But it's nearby, so you might as well color it, too.

CIRCUMCISION

Figure 2 shows a *circumcised* penis. *Circumcision* is an operation that removes the *foreskin* of the penis. The *foreskin* is part of the special skin covering of the penis. The operation is usually done when a baby is only a few days old.

Most males in this country have been circumcised. But there are also many who still have their foreskins. If a boy has not been circumcised, his foreskin covers most or all of the glans.

When a male baby is born, the foreskin and glans are usually attached. Sooner or later, the foreskin works itself free. By the time a boy becomes an adult, if not sooner, he can retract the foreskin. This means he can pull it back over the glans and down the shaft of the penis, as shown in Figure 3.

You may be wondering why people have their sons circumcised. Maybe you have other questions about the operation. If so, you'll find more information about circumcision in Chapter 8.

---

pubic (PEW-bik)
anus (AY-nus)
feces (FEE-sees)
bowel (BOW-uhl)
circumcised (SIR-kum-sized)
circumcision (sir-kum-SISH-un)
foreskin (FOUR-skin)

By the time the class has colored in the different parts, I've said the word "penis" out loud about twenty-eight times. Everyone is used to my saying this and other words that aren't usually said out loud in classrooms. My students no longer have to go crazy each time I use these words. Besides, the pictures look funny. Everyone is laughing. Laughter makes it easier to deal with embarrassed or nervous feelings.

I have another reason for getting the kids to color these drawings. It helps them to remember the names of these organs. If

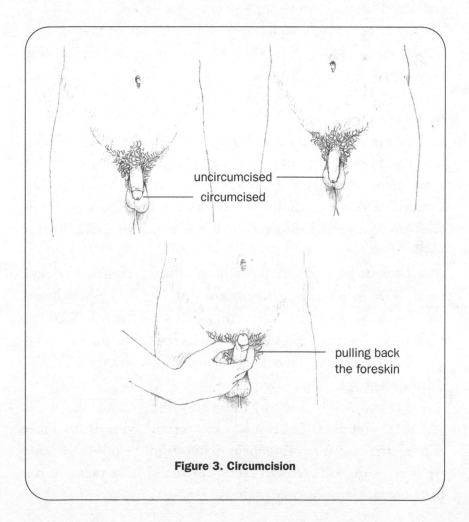

uncircumcised

circumcised

pulling back
the foreskin

Figure 3. Circumcision

you just look at the drawing, the names of the parts may not stick in your mind. If you spend time coloring the parts, you have to pay attention. You're more likely to remember their names. These are important parts of the body. It's worth a little effort to learn their names.

While everyone is coloring, we talk about slang words. People don't always use the medical names for these body parts. They sometimes use slang words.

The boys in the back row of my very first puberty class were walking dictionaries of slang. Whenever I said "penis" or "vagina" out loud, their brains would buzz and hum with dozens of slang words. It was too much for them to keep to themselves. Leaning out of their seats, they flapped their arms, playfully punching each other. Gleefully, they whispered and hissed these so-called dirty words at one another.

In the end, the thrill of saying these "bad" words out loud proved too much for the boys. The entire back row dissolved into fits of wild giggling. Some of them were actually rolling around on the floor. Soon, the entire class was totally out of control. "Maybe," I thought, "I'm not cut out for this line of work."

I might have given up teaching puberty classes then and there, but I had a sudden brainstorm. I turned to the blackboard and started to list all the slang words that were flying around the classroom. I encouraged the whole class to add to the list. Soon the blackboard was covered with slang words, and the class was calm enough for us to go on.

I'm not exactly sure why this works, but over the years, I've learned that it does. The best way to keep these words from disrupting the class is to bring them right out in the open. So while we're coloring, kids call out slang words and I list them on the blackboard. Here are some of them.

SOME SLANG WORDS FOR
THE PENIS AND TESTICLES

PENIS			TESTICLES	
cock	peter	tool	balls	cojones
dick	dong	frankfurter	nuts	things
prick	dingus	thing	eggs	bangers
schlong	dork	pecker	rocks	hangers
wee-wee	meat	dinky	jewels	stones
wanger	pisser	penie	cubes	seeds

After we've listed them on the board, the class talks about these slang words. We discuss which words we'd use with a friend, with a doctor, or with our moms. We also talk about people's reactions to slang words. Some people object to these words. They may get upset if they hear you using them. You may or may not care about upsetting people in this way. But you should at least be aware that many people find slang words offensive.

THE FEMALE SEX ORGANS

When everyone finishes coloring the male sex organs, they color the female sex organs. The sex organs on the outside of a woman's body are called the vulva. The vulva has several parts. At the top is a pad of fatty tissue called the *mons*. Wiry, curly pubic hair covers the mons in grown women. I tell the class to color the mons and the pubic hair red.

Next, we move toward the bottom of the mons. There it divides into two folds of skin called the outer lips. I suggest blue polka dots for the outer lips. Between the outer lips lie the two inner lips. You might try red stripes for the inner lips.

---

mons (MONZ)

The inner lips join at the top. The folds of skin where the lips join form a sort of hood. In Figure 2, you can see the tip of the *clitoris* peeking out from under this hood. The rest of the clitoris lies under the skin where you can't see it. Color the tip of the clitoris blue.

Straight down from the clitoris is the urinary opening. This is where urine leaves a woman's body. I tell the class to circle it with red.

Below the urinary opening is the *vaginal* opening. It leads to the vagina inside the body. The vagina connects the outside of the body to the sex organs inside a woman's body. I suggest circling the vaginal opening with blue. (People often use the word "vagina" when they should say "vulva." The vagina is inside the body. "Vulva" is the correct term for the sex organs on the outside of the female body.) Finally, we come to the anus. Color it any way you like.

While they're coloring the female genitals, we also make a list of slang words for these parts of a woman's body.

SOME SLANG WORDS FOR
THE CLITORIS, VULVA, AND VAGINA

CLITORIS	VULVA AND VAGINA		
clit	pussy	box	snatch
bud	cunt	beaver	poontang
pea	muff	honeypot	pudie
man in the boat	stuff	hole	slit
spot	quim	thing	twat

By the time they've colored the sex organs and made lists of slang words, everyone has giggled off a good deal of nervous

---

clitoris (KLIT-or-iss)
vaginal (VAJ-in-uhl)

energy and embarrassment. They've also gotten a good idea of where these body parts are. This helps in understanding how babies are made.

SEXUAL INTERCOURSE

Sexual intercourse between a male and a female can make a baby. When a male and female have intercourse, the penis fits inside the vagina. As soon as I tell my class this, they always have two questions right off the bat. First, they want to know *how* a penis can get inside a vagina.

I begin my answer by explaining about *erections*. Sometimes, the penis gets stiff and hard and sticks out from the body at an angle. (See Figure 4.) This is called having an erection. Males of all ages, even babies, have erections. An erection can happen when a male is having sexual feelings and at other times, too. During an

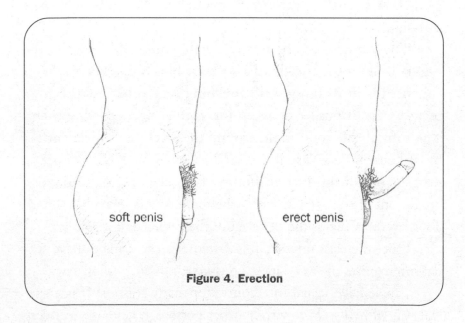

soft penis   erect penis

Figure 4. Erection

erections (ih-REK-shuns)

erection the tissue inside the penis fills with blood. This tissue has millions of tiny spaces. Usually, the spaces are empty and the penis is limp and soft. When a male has an erection, these spaces fill with so much blood that the tissue becomes stiff and hard. The penis swells, becomes erect, and stands out from the body. Some people call an erection a "boner" or a "hard-on." The penis can get so stiff and hard it feels like there's a bone in there. There isn't any bone, though, just blood-filled tissue.

If a couple wants to have intercourse, they get close enough together for the erect penis to be able to enter the vagina. They press their bodies together and move so the penis slides back and forth in the vagina, giving them sexual pleasure.

You might think it would be difficult for the penis to enter the vagina. After all, the vaginal opening isn't very large. However, the vaginal opening is *very* elastic and can stretch to many times its usual size. In fact, the vaginal opening is so elastic that when a woman gives birth, it can stretch enough to allow a baby to pass through.

The vagina is a tube of soft, pliable muscle. Normally the vagina is like a balloon that hasn't been blown up. The vagina is collapsed with its inner walls touching each other. As the erect penis enters, it pushes between the vaginal walls, parting them. The soft, pliable walls mold around the erect penis for a perfect fit. When a male is sexually excited ("turned on"), he produces a drop or two of fluid from the tip of his erect penis. Fluid also comes out of the vaginal walls when a female is sexually excited. This "wetness" helps the penis enter the vagina comfortably.

Once the class understands *how* males and females have sexual intercourse, the next question is *why*.

People have sexual intercourse for many reasons. It is a special way of being close with another person. It can also feel very good. Some kids in my class find this hard to believe. But the sex organs have many nerve endings. These nerve endings send messages to pleasure centers in our brains. Stroking these parts of our bodies or rubbing them in the right ways can give us good feelings all over our bodies. Another reason men and women have sexual intercourse is to make a baby. But babies don't start to grow every time a male and a female have intercourse, just sometimes.

MAKING BABIES

To make a baby an *ovum* from the female and a *sperm* from the male must come together. This can happen as a result of sexual intercourse.

Sometimes a woman's ovum is called her "egg," and a man's sperm is called his "seed." These terms confuse some of the boys and girls in my class. To them, seeds are what we plant in the ground to grow flowers or vegetables. And eggs are what chickens lay. But an ovum and a sperm are not like these kinds of eggs and seeds.

For starters, an ovum is much smaller than the eggs we cook for breakfast. In fact, it is smaller than the smallest dot you could make with the tip of even the sharpest pencil. A sperm is even smaller. You could think of a sperm as half a seed and an ovum as the other half. When these two halves come together, a human baby begins to grow. Actually, the sperm and the ovum are cells. Our bodies are made of billions and billions of cells. There are many different types of cells. But the ovum and the sperm are the only kind of cells that can join together to make a single cell. From this single cell, a baby grows.

---

ovum (OH-vum)
sperm (SPURM)

Sperm and Ejaculation

Sperm are made in the testicles, the two egg-shaped organs inside the scrotum. They are stored in hollow tubes called sperm *ducts*. A boy's testicles begin making sperm during puberty. They usually continue making new sperm every day for the rest of his life.

When he's having sex, a male may *ejaculate*. During ejaculation, muscles in the sex organs contract. These contractions pump sperm up into the main part of the body. There, they mix with other fluids. This mixture is a creamy, white fluid called *semen*. Muscle contractions pump the semen through the *urethra*, the hollow tube that runs the length of the penis. The semen then spurts out the opening in the tip of the penis. (See Figure 5.)

On average, less than a teaspoon of semen comes out of the penis during an ejaculation. This small amount of semen contains millions of sperm! During sex, a male may ejaculate between 300 and 500 million sperm into the female's vagina. Some of these sperm make their way to the top of the vagina. There, they enter a tiny tunnel that leads into the *uterus,* or *womb*. (See Figure 6.) The uterus is the place inside a woman's body where a baby develops.

Some of the sperm then swim to the top of the uterus and into one of the two uterine tubes. Many sperm never make it as far as the uterus. They get lost in the vagina. Other sperm get lost in the uterus. The sperm that get lost and don't make it are eventually dissolved by the woman's body.

Of the millions of sperm ejaculated into the vagina, only a few make it to the top of the uterus and from there into the

---

ducts (DUKTS)
ejaculate (ih-JACK-you-late)
semen (SEE-mun)
urethra (you-REE-thruh)
uterus (YOU-ter-us)
womb (WOOM) rhymes with "room"

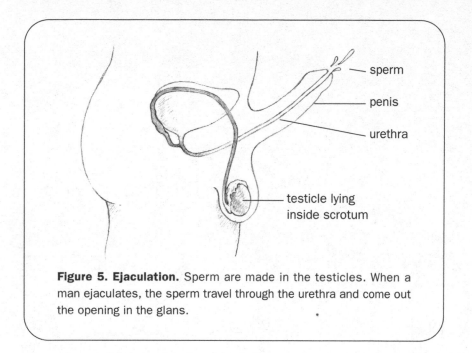

sperm

penis

urethra

testicle lying
inside scrotum

Figure 5. Ejaculation. Sperm are made in the testicles. When a man ejaculates, the sperm travel through the urethra and come out the opening in the glans.

uterine, or Fallopian, tubes. These are two tubes that connect to the upper part of the uterus on either side. Here, inside one of these tubes, the sperm may meet and join together with an ovum.

Ovum and Ovulation

A girl is born with hundreds of thousands of *ova.* ("Ova" is the plural form of "ovum." If you're talking about more than one ovum, you say "ova.") Ova are stored in two organs called *ovaries.* A young girl's ova are not mature. The first ovum doesn't ripen until she is well into puberty.

A grown woman usually produces a ripe ovum from one of her ovaries about once a month. When it is fully mature, the ripe

uterine (YOU-ter-in)
ova (OH-vuh)
ovaries (OH-vuh-reez)

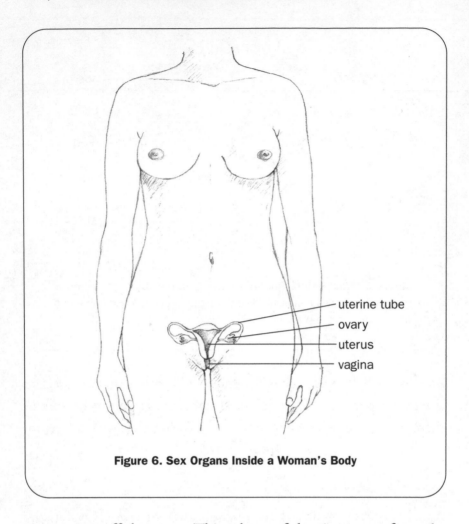

Figure 6. Sex Organs Inside a Woman's Body

ovum pops off the *ovary*. This release of the ripe ovum from the ovary is called *ovulation*. (See Figure 7.)

After it pops off the ovary, the ovum enters one of the uterine tubes. The ends of the uterine tube reach out and sweep the ovum into the tube. Tiny hairs inside the tube wave back and forth. Slowly, their gentle waving helps move the ovum through the tube.

---

ovary (OH-vuh-ree)
ovulation (ahv-you-LAY-shun)

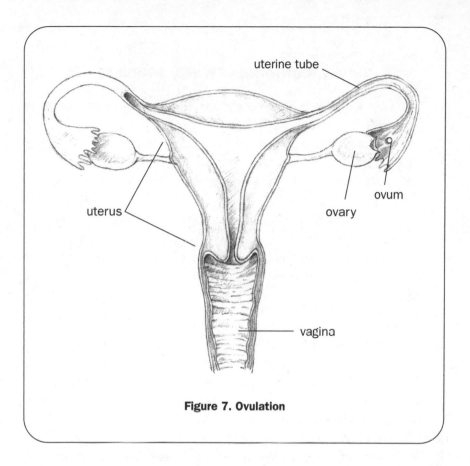

Figure 7. Ovulation

Fertilization, Pregnancy, and Birth

As the ovum travels through the tube, it may meet some sperm. If so, one of the sperm may enter the ovum. This joining of an ovum and a sperm is called *fertilization*.

The ovum can be *fertilized* by a sperm only during the first twenty-four hours after it leaves the ovary. But sperm can stay alive inside the female body for up to five days. This means fertilization is possible if a male and female have sex on the day of ovu-

fertilization (fur-tuh-iz-AY-shun)
fertilized ovary (FUR-tuh-lized OH-vuh-ree)

TWINS, CONJOINED TWINS, TRIPLETS . . .

As soon as I explain about fertilization, hands shoot up all around the classroom.

"What if more than one sperm fertilizes the egg? Will the woman have twins?"

I explain that it's only possible for one sperm to enter an ovum and fertilize it. The instant a sperm begins to enter, the ovum goes through chemical changes. These changes make it impossible for another sperm to enter.

But that's usually just the beginning of the questions. Although it would take another whole book to answer all the questions, here are some basic facts to help satisfy your curiosity.

- *Fraternal* twins are one of the two types of twins. (See Figure 9.) Fraternal twins happen when there are two ova, each fertilized by a different sperm. Usually a woman's ovary produces only one ripe ovum at a time, but once in a while the ovary produces two ripe ova at the same time. Each of these ova could then be fertilized by a different sperm. If both fertilized ova plant themselves in the lining of the uterus, the woman will be pregnant with fraternal twins. Such twins may not look alike. They may not even be the same sex.

- *Identical* twins develop from a single fertilized ovum that splits in two. (See Figure 10.) The splitting happens soon after the fertilization. No one knows why. Because identical twins come from the same ovum and sperm, they look alike. They are always the same sex.

- When twins are born, one baby comes out first. The other baby usually comes out a few minutes later. Sometimes more time passes before the second twin is born. There have even been cases where a whole day passed between the births of the first and second twin.

---

fraternal (fruh-TURN-ull)
identical (eye-DEN-tih-kull)

- It is possible for a woman to give birth to fraternal twins who have two different fathers. For this to happen, the woman would have to have sex with two different men right around the time she ovulates.

- *Conjoined,* or *Siamese,* twins are identical twins who are born with their bodies attached to each other in some way. For some unknown reason, the fertilized ovum doesn't split completely. The babies develop with parts of their bodies joined together.

  Identical twins are pretty rare. Conjoined twins are much rarer. Conjoined twins may be joined in a number of ways. If they are joined at the feet, the shoulders, or the arms, an operation can separate the babies. In other cases, it's more difficult to separate them. They may be joined in such a way that cutting them apart would kill one or both. For instance, the bodies may be joined at the chest and share one heart. Some parents decide to have the operation done even if one baby may die. Other parents decide against the operation. If they aren't separated, the twins spend their lives attached.

- Triplets (three babies), quadruplets (four), quintuplets (five), sextuplets (six), septuplets (seven), and octuplets (eight) happen even less often than twins. When more than three babies are born at one time, the chance of all the babies surviving is low. Because there are so many of them, they're much smaller than normal babies and are born before they develop fully. As far as we know, the largest number of babies born at one time is twelve. But some of them died. There was a case in Iowa where a woman gave birth to seven babies, all of whom survived. Not too long after that, eight live babies were born to a couple in Texas, but one of them died shortly after birth.

Women who give birth to more than two babies at one time are usually taking special medicines to get pregnant. Because these women have had problems getting pregnant in the past, their doctors put them on drugs to stimulate the ovaries. But such drugs often stimulate the ovaries too much, so that several ripe ova are released at the same time.

Conjoined (kun-JOINED)
Siamese (sigh-uh-MEEZ)

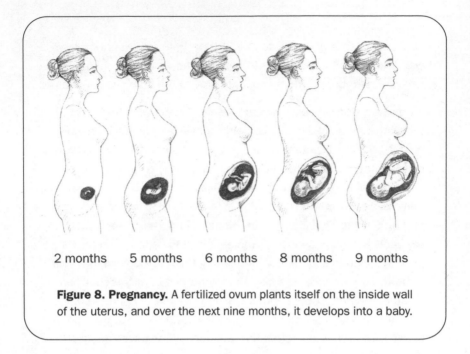

2 months   5 months   6 months   8 months   9 months

Figure 8. Pregnancy. A fertilized ovum plants itself on the inside wall of the uterus, and over the next nine months, it develops into a baby.

lation or on any of the five days before ovulation. Most times, the ovum travels through the uterine tube into the uterus without meeting a sperm. A few days after it reaches the uterus, the unfertilized ovum breaks down. If the ovum has been fertilized, it doesn't break down. Once it gets to the uterus, it plants itself there, and, over the next nine months, it grows into a baby.

The uterus is a hollow organ. In a grown woman, the uterus is normally the size of a pear. But the thick, muscular walls of the uterus are very elastic. This allows the uterus to expand during pregnancy. (See Figure 8.)

When the baby is ready to come out, the mother's uterus begins to contract. The tiny tunnel connecting the uterus to the vagina stretches open. Powerful contractions push the baby out of the uterus and into the vagina. The contractions continue. The baby is pushed through the vagina, then out the vaginal opening, and into the world. Hello, baby!

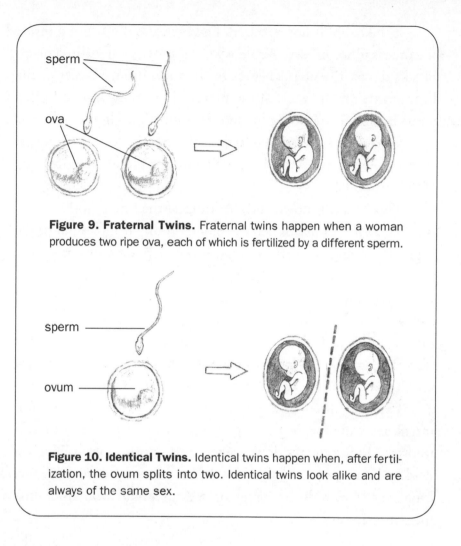

Figure 9. Fraternal Twins. Fraternal twins happen when a woman produces two ripe ova, each of which is fertilized by a different sperm.

Figure 10. Identical Twins. Identical twins happen when, after fertilization, the ovum splits into two. Identical twins look alike and are always of the same sex.

MENSTRUATION

Each month, as the ovary gets ready to release a ripe ovum, the uterus prepares itself. If the ovum is fertilized, it will plant itself in the tissue lining the uterus. The fertilized ovum will need plenty of rich blood and nourishment as it develops. So, as the ovum is ripening in the ovary, the lining of the uterus grows thicker. It develops new blood vessels and spongy, blood-filled tissue that will nourish the ovum if it's fertilized.

If the ovum is not fertilized, however, the thick lining inside the uterus is not needed. About a week after the unfertilized ovum breaks down, the uterus begins to shed the lining. Pieces of the lining slide off the walls of the uterus. The spongy, blood-filled tissue breaks down, becoming mostly liquid. This liquid, which is called the *menstrual* flow, collects in the bottom of the uterus. It then slowly dribbles into the vagina and out the vaginal opening. (See Figure 11.)

This breaking down and shedding of the lining of the uterus is called *menstruation*. When the bloody lining dribbles out of the vaginal opening, we say a woman is *menstruating*, or *having her period*.

The amount of blood that dribbles out during a period varies. All together, there's usually one-quarter to one-third cup of menstrual flow. It doesn't come out all at once. It dribbles out slowly, then it stops. It may take only a couple of days or it may take a week or so for all of the menstrual flow to leave the body.

Once the bleeding stops, the uterus starts growing a new lining to get ready for the next ripe ovum. If that ovum is not fertilized, the lining breaks down again, and another period begins. And so it goes, month after month, for much of a woman's life. One exception is during pregnancy. A pregnant woman doesn't menstruate.

When will you get your first period? No one can say for sure, but this book will help you make an educated guess. In the chapters that follow, we'll talk more about menstruation, your first period, and the other physical and emotional changes of puberty.

---

menstrual (MEN-stroo-uhl)
menstruation (men-stroo-AY-shun)
menstruating (MEN-stroo-ay-ting)

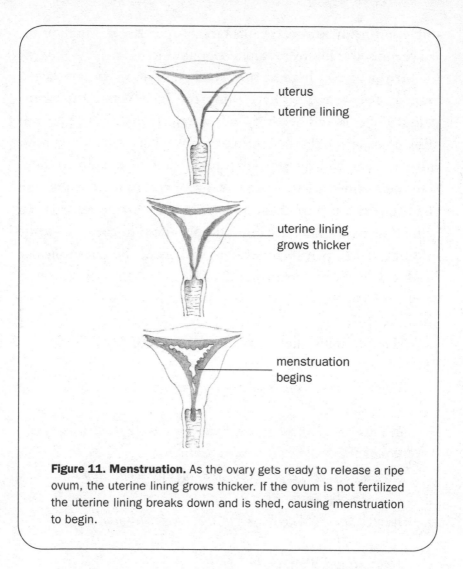

uterus
uterine lining

uterine lining grows thicker

menstruation begins

Figure 11. Menstruation. As the ovary gets ready to release a ripe ovum, the uterine lining grows thicker. If the ovum is not fertilized the uterine lining breaks down and is shed, causing menstruation to begin.

EVERYTHING YOU EVER WANTED TO KNOW . . .

If you're like the girls in our classes and workshops, you have lots of questions about what's happening to your body. It isn't always easy to ask these questions. We may feel too embarrassed. We may think our questions are too dumb. We may be afraid that everyone else already knows the answers. Maybe they'll laugh at us. Maybe they'll think we're stupid or "out of it."

If you've ever felt like this, you're not alone. In my classes, we play a game called "Everything You Ever Wanted to Know About Puberty and Sex but Were Afraid to Ask." We pass out slips of paper at the beginning of class. The kids write their questions and put the slips in a special box. They don't have to sign their names. I am the only one who gets to see the question slips. The box is locked and it stays in the classroom. Kids can write down questions any time and put them in the box. At the end of class, I open the question box. I read the questions out loud and do my best to answer them. If I don't know the answer, I say so. Then I make a point of trying to find the answer before the next class.

Here are some questions from our question box:

What if you lied and said you got your period, but really you didn't?

Is it okay to wear a bra even though you don't really need one?

What's that gooey stuff on my underpants?

How do you get people to stop making comments about your breasts?

What is the right age for a girl to grow breasts and get pubic hair?

How tall will I be?

What if I get my period at school?

Does having your period hurt?

How do I tell my mom I want a bra?

Which is better for girls to use—tampons or pads?

What's the best stuff to buy for pimples?

One breast is growing, but the other one is completely flat. Will I be lopsided?

READING THIS BOOK

This book answers these and other questions from our class question box, our workshops, and our readers. You may want to read this book with your parents, with a friend, or by yourself. You may want to read it straight through from beginning to end. Or, perhaps, you'll jump around, reading a chapter here and there. However you read this book, we hope that you'll enjoy it. We hope, too, that you'll learn as much from reading it as we did from writing it.

2.

YOUR BREASTS: AN OWNER'S MANUAL

I no longer remember when I first noticed my breasts were developing. I *do* remember the first time someone else noticed. I was baby-sitting seven-year-old twin girls. It was the first time I ever sat for these girls. (It was also the last time. They dumped their pet guppies into the toilet—"so the guppies would have more room to swim around." While I was on my hands and knees, fishing guppies out of the toilet bowl, they were at work in the kitchen. The little dears put their miniature turtle into the toaster—"to warm it up.")

The evening got off to a bad start. They were nice as pie while their mom and dad were still there. As soon as the door closed behind their parents, they jumped on me.

"You've got titties. Let us see, let us see," they demanded, pulling open my blouse. "We can't wait till we get titties," they shrieked.

I finally managed to get the two of them off me and to button up my blouse. I had never been so embarrassed in my life!

You may be as eager as those twins or as mortified as I was. Either way, sooner or later your breasts will begin to develop.

Breast development is often the first sign of puberty. This isn't always the case, though. For many girls, pubic hair is the first sign. For some girls, underarm hair comes first. Sometimes breast development, pubic hair, and/or underarm hair all start at the same time. Whether or not breast development is your first sign, at some point during puberty, your breasts will begin to develop.

THE BREAST

On each breast, you have a *nipple* and *areola*. The *nipple* is the raised nub in the center of each breast. It may be light pink, dark brown, or any color in between. The *areola* is the colored ring of flesh around the nipple. (See Figure 12.)

The nipple and areola are very sensitive. Cold temperatures, touching, and sexual feelings can make them *erect. Erect* means the nipple gets stiff and "stands up." The areola may pucker up and get bumpy. These changes are temporary. After a while, the nipple and areola return to normal.

During childhood, only the nipple is raised. The rest of the breast is flat and smooth. During puberty, the breasts begin to swell and to stand out from the chest more.

Inside the Breast

Figure 13 shows the inside of a grown woman's breast. The breast has a good deal of fat tissue. There are also milk glands and ducts.

---

nipple (NIP-puhl)
areola (ah-REE-oh-luh)

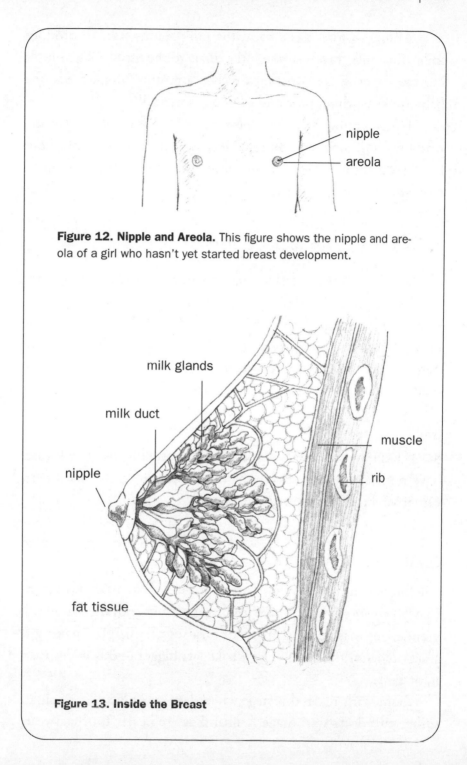

Figure 12. Nipple and Areola. This figure shows the nipple and areola of a girl who hasn't yet started breast development.

Figure 13. Inside the Breast

After a woman has a baby, the milk glands start to produce milk. The milk travels through the ducts to the nipple. The nipple has twenty or so tiny openings. When a mother breast-feeds, the baby sucks on the nipple and out comes the milk.

During puberty, your breasts develop. Your body is getting ready for a time when you may decide to have a baby. But your breasts are not yet ready to make milk; that doesn't happen until a woman actually gives birth.

FIVE STAGES OF BREAST DEVELOPMENT

As you grow from a girl to a woman, your breasts grow and develop. Doctors divide breast growth into five stages. Figure 14 shows the five stages. Read the descriptions of these stages in the next pages. Then compare your body to the drawings of the five stages. See if you can figure out the stage you are in.

Stage 1: Childhood

Stage 1 is the childhood stage, before puberty begins. The breasts have not started to develop. The nipples are the only raised part. Otherwise, the breasts are flat.

Stage 2: Breast Buds Develop

The breasts start to develop during Stage 2. A small, flat, button-like *breast bud* forms under each nipple. It contains fat, milk glands, and tissue. The breast bud raises the nipple, making it stick out from the chest. The areola gets bigger and is wider than in Stage 1.

Some girls reach this stage when they are only seven or eight. Other girls don't start Stage 2 until they are nearly fourteen years

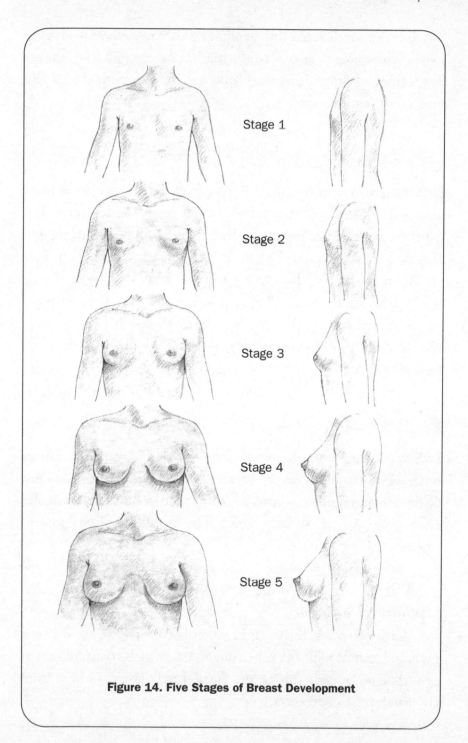

Figure 14. Five Stages of Breast Development

old, but most girls reach this stage when they're eight and a half to eleven years old. (For more information on ages and stages, see pages 65–69.) Stage 2 may last from a matter of months to a year and a half or more.

Stage 3: Development Continues

Breast development continues during Stage 3. The breasts become larger. The areolas also continue to get bigger. They stand out more from the chest. You may notice that the nipples, too, are getting larger. In this stage, the breasts are adult in shape, but they are smaller than they will be when you are an adult.

Girls usually reach this stage when they're ten to thirteen years old, but some girls reach Stage 3 when they're younger than ten or older than thirteen. Stage 3 may last a few months or as long as two years.

Stage 4: Nipple and Areola Form Mound

In Stage 4, the areola and nipple continue to enlarge. They form a separate little mound on the breast. They stick out above the rest of the breast. Figure 15 shows the difference in the nipple and areola in Stage 3, Stage 4, and Stage 5. The breasts are often "pointy" or cone-shaped in Stage 4.

Some girls skip Stage 4 and go directly to Stage 5. Some never develop beyond Stage 4. Still other girls develop a raised mound again in Stage 5.

Girls often reach this stage when they're twelve to fourteen years old, but as with the other stages, many girls reach Stage 4 at ages that are outside this range. Stage 4 may last anywhere from eight months to two years.

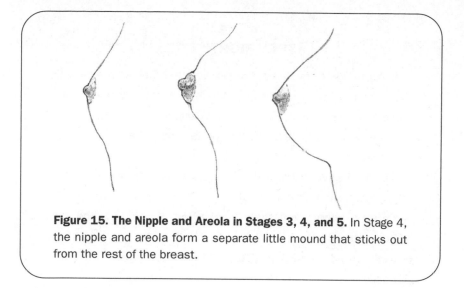

Figure 15. The Nipple and Areola in Stages 3, 4, and 5. In Stage 4, the nipple and areola form a separate little mound that sticks out from the rest of the breast.

Stage 5: Adult

In Stage 5, the nipple and areola no longer form a separate mound on the breast. (Again, see Figure 15.) This is the adult stage. The breasts are fully developed. However, some girls' breasts do continue to grow somewhat even after they've reached this stage.

Even though the breasts have reached their adult size, they may not be very large. In fact, some grown women have breasts smaller than the ones shown here. (We'll talk more about breast size in the next few pages.)

Most girls reach Stage 5 between the ages of thirteen and sixteen, but some girls reach this stage when they're younger than thirteen and others when they're older than sixteen.

Timing and Rate of Development

The time it takes for breasts to develop fully is different for different girls. Some girls begin Stage 2 and within eighteen months

THE "RIGHT" AGE

Some girls get to feeling down because their bodies are slow to develop. They're eager to have breasts and mature bodies. Their classmates are developing while they still look "like little kids." Other girls are upset because they're developing earlier than their classmates.

Girls often worry that they're not developing at the "right" age. But there isn't one "right" age. Girls start to develop at a wide range of different ages. A girl's body develops at the age that's right for her. If you're worried about being early or late to develop, read the section "Starting Puberty: Ages and Stages" on pages 65–69.

If you're bothered because you're developing early, remember, the other girls will catch up to you. If you're unhappy because your body isn't changing as fast as you'd like, remember, the changes *will* happen eventually. Then you'll wonder what all the fuss was about!

they are entering Stage 5. Other girls take over six years to go from Stage 2 to Stage 5. On the average, breast development takes three to five years.

People often think girls who start to develop earlier than their classmates also develop faster than other girls their age, but *when* you start to develop has no effect on *how fast* you develop. Just because a girl starts first doesn't mean she'll finish first.

When you start to develop is not related to *how big* your breasts will be when you are fully grown, either. An early starter may wind up having large, medium, or small breasts. The same is true for girls who are late starters and for those who start at an average age.

Breast Stages and Your First Period

Most girls have their first menstrual period while they are in Stage 3 or 4 of breast development. However, some girls don't have their period until Stage 5. There are even few girls who have their first period in Stage 2, though this is rare. If you have any bleeding before you develop either breast buds or pubic hair, you need to see a doctor and get it checked out.

BREAST SIZE

Imagine a gym full of girls standing with their arms held at shoulder level, elbows bent. Jerking their elbows back and forth to a one-two, one-two count, they chant:

> *We must, we must,*
> *We must increase our busts.*
> *It's better, it's better,*
> *It's better for the sweater.*
> *We may, we may,*
> *We may get big someday.*

That was gym class in the "good old days." We hope girls no longer have to do this. Not that there's anything wrong with the exercise. It's good for toning and firming the muscles of the chest wall. If you do this exercise a lot, the chest muscles underneath the breast will get thicker. This may make your breasts stand out more, but it won't make your breasts larger. Your breasts are mostly glands and fat tissue. No amount of exercise will enlarge them.

Although the exercise itself is fine, the chant is not. All that business about "we must increase our busts" puts such emphasis on having big breasts. It's as if big breasts were somehow better than small ones. Small breasts do as good a job of making breast milk as large ones. Small breasts give us the same pleasurable feelings when they are stroked or touched. Small breasts are just as beautiful as big ones. It's like the difference between being blonde and brunette. Some people prefer one look, some people prefer the other.

However, there are so many big-busted, glamorous women in advertisements, films, and TV shows that it's easy to get the idea that big breasts are more womanly or more sexy than small ones. You'd be surprised how many people don't feel that way. Besides, anyone who decides whether to like you based on breast size isn't a person worth knowing.

Still, we do live in a country that has a hang-up about breasts. Some women with small breasts feel unhappy about their bodies. Some even have operations to enlarge their breasts.

Breast size can be a problem for large-breasted women, too. In some cases, the breasts are so large that their size affects posture and causes back pains. There are also operations to reduce breasts to a more comfortable size.

CONCERNS ABOUT DEVELOPING BREASTS

Could a girl's breasts burst?
Could a girl's boobs pop like a balloon?

The answer to these questions is, "No." For a long time, we didn't understand what was behind these questions. Then one day, a girl in our class clued us in:

Grown-ups are always saying things like, "Oh, you're really popping out," or "You're sure bursting out all over." Sometimes my breasts feel sore, like they really are about to burst, so I wondered.

—SUSAN, AGE 11

If you've worried about this, you can stop worrying. Your breasts won't pop or burst. Many girls we talked to had concerns or worries about their developing breasts. In the next few pages, we'll share their concerns with you.

Itchy, Tender, Sore, or Painful Breasts

One or both of your developing breasts may be itchy, tender, sore, or downright painful at times. One girl told us:

> I was really freaked out. I had these little flat bumps under my nipples. They hurt all the time, especially if they got hit or something. They were so sore. I thought maybe something was wrong.
>
> —KAREN, AGE 11

Developing breasts are often itchy, sore, tender, or even painful. This is not a sign that something is wrong. It's just a normal part of growing up. The discomfort usually goes away on its own. The pain usually isn't severe. In the rare cases when the pain is severe, the girl should see her doctor. He or she can prescribe drugs to help the problem. Once a girl's periods begin, she may find that her breasts are sore around the time of her menstrual period. For more information on this, see Chapter 6.

Breast Lumps

A breast bud feels like a small button under the nipple. Girls sometime mistake them for the breast lumps that are a sign of cancer, but breast cancer never affects girls whose breasts are just starting to develop. Older girls sometimes have problems with lumpy breasts around the time of their periods. (For more infor-

PROTECTING YOUR BREASTS

Breast cancer is rarely, if ever, found in teenagers. But what you eat during these years may affect your chances of developing breast cancer later in life.

Why? Because between puberty and the time of a woman's first pregnancy, cells in the breast are still maturing. During this time, the breasts are especially vulnerable to the harmful effects of cancer-causing substances in the diet and the environment. A young woman's exposure to these harmful substances can lead to cancer many years later.

Scientists still don't know exactly what causes breast cancer. But a diet high in fat (especially animal fat) may increase your chances of developing breast cancer. Likewise, drinking alcohol may increase the risk.

On the other hand, a high-fiber diet with lots of fruits and vegetables (especially leafy green vegetables) may lower the risk. Regular exercise may also lower your chances of developing breast cancer.

You'll find more information on healthy diet and exercise in Chapter 4. Follow the advice there and help protect your breasts at this important time in your life.

mation on this, see pages 146–147.) However, lumps under the nipple in girls just starting puberty are perfectly normal, just another part of growing up.

Uneven Size or Rate of Development

Some girls worry because one breast develops before the other. One girl told us:

One of my breasts was starting to grow. The other one was still completely flat. I was afraid that the other one would never grow—that I was only going to have one breast instead of two.

—MIAYSHA, AGE 14

Other girls worry because one breast is larger than the other:

Both of mine started growing at the same time, but one of mine was a lot bigger than the other one. I was worried that I was going to grow up all lopsided.

—ROSIE, AGE 14

Often a breast bud develops under one nipple while the other breast remains flat. The second breast bud usually develops within six to twelve months.

While a girl is developing, one breast may be noticeably larger than the other. This is perfectly normal. It is most common in Stages 2 to 4. By the time a girl reaches Stage 5, the two breasts are usually about the same size, but some girls continue to have a noticeable difference in size even as adults. If the difference in size bothers a woman, she can wear a padded bra or bra insert (see page 49), or she can have plastic surgery to correct the size difference. However, this surgery usually isn't done until a girl has finished puberty. In the meantime, she can wear a padded bra or bra insert.

Inverted Nipples

One girl described this condition:

---

inverted (in-VUR-ted)

One of my nipples didn't stick out. The other did. It sort of puckered in. I wondered why.

—DIANA, AGE 16

This girl is describing an *inverted* nipple. In this condition, one or both nipples point inward. They sink into the areola instead of pointing out. (See Figure 16.) Often this condition is present at birth, but it may not become obvious until puberty. As the breasts develop, the inverted nipple may start to point out, or it may not. There are also women who have "shy" nipples. One or both of their nipples become inverted for a while when stimulated.

You may have heard that a woman with inverted nipples can't breast-feed her baby. This is not true. Many women with inverted nipples breast-feed their babies, in some cases with the help of a simple plastic shield.

Inverted nipples may be prone to infection. It's important to keep them clean. If you're not sure how to clean an inverted nipple, ask your doctor or school nurse for advice. After puberty, if a nipple suddenly becomes inverted, you should see a doctor. This doesn't always mean something is wrong, but it should be checked

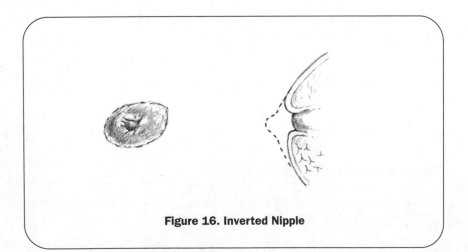

Figure 16. Inverted Nipple

out by a doctor. Other than this, inverted nipples usually are not a cause for concern.

Nipple Discharge

Some girls worry because they have a *nipple discharge*—fluid coming from one or both nipples. A nipple discharge that comes out only if the nipple is squeezed and appears only occasionally is usually normal. The fluid is made by the body to keep the breast ducts clear. It is usually white, clear, or slightly yellow-green.

Most nipple discharges are nothing to worry about. However, nipple discharge can be a sign of a medical problem, so a doctor should check out nipple discharge in a girl or a young woman. (By the way, don't squeeze your nipples to try to produce the discharge. The act of squeezing can actually cause your breasts to produce more discharge.)

BRAS

When should a girl start wearing a bra?
Does a girl even need to wear a bra at all?

There are no set answers to these questions. You have to decide for yourself. Some girls wear a bra for comfort. The bra supports their breasts and keeps them from "jiggling." Others wear bras because they feel self-conscious without one. Some wear bras because they're afraid their breasts will droop or sag. Actually, sagging results from fat tissue replacing milk ducts and glands as we age. No bra can prevent this. Pregnancy and breast-feeding can enlarge and stretch the breasts. This adds to sagging. (You may have seen pictures of the sagging breasts of elderly women in magazines like *National Geographic*. Malnutrition and other factors, not lack of a bra, cause this sagging.)

We often hear from girls who would like to wear a bra although they don't really "need" one. One girl wrote:

> I'm eleven years old. . . . I'm not very big. In fact, I'm kind of flat. Do you think it is silly for me to want a bra?
>
> —AUDREY, AGE 11

There's nothing silly about wearing a bra, no matter how "flat" you are. If you're teased about wearing a bra you don't really need, you could say:

- Oh, I'm just getting used to wearing one.

- I like them better than undershirts.

- I feel more comfortable this way.

Some girls tell us they are embarrassed to ask their parents for a bra. We tell them to ask anyway. Your parents may be waiting for *you* to bring the topic up. *They* might be afraid they'd embarrass *you!* You could say:

- Would it be okay with you if I wore a bra?

- When do you think I should start wearing a bra?

- How old were you when you started to wear a bra?

You could also write a note explaining how you feel. Your parents might say, "Oh, don't be silly, you don't need a bra yet." If so, you could say:

- Well, maybe not, but I'd *like* one anyway.

- I'd feel more comfortable wearing one.

Buying a Bra

Bras are sold just about everywhere these days. Some department stores and stores such as Kmart and Sears usually have a fitter. She's a saleswoman who has special training in fitting bras. She can help you select the size and type of bra that's right for you. The service is free. You don't have to buy anything. It's silly not to take advantage of this "freebie."

Training Bras and Fitted Bras

Training bras, despite their name, do not train your breasts to grow. Some training bras have flat or nearly flat cups. This type is a good choice if you've only just started to develop. They are also good if you haven't started to develop, but would still like to wear a bra.

Some training bras, and most regular bras, are fitted bras. This means they come in different sizes—for example, 28AAA, 34B, 44D. Bra sizes are made up of two parts:

- BAND SIZE: This is a number, usually between 28 and 44. The band size is also called the body size. It tells the number of inches around your body at breast level.

- CUP SIZE: This is given in letters: AAA, AA, A, B, C, D, DD, E, and EE. Triple A (AAA) is the smallest cup size. Double E (EE) is the largest.

Sizing Yourself Up

Before you go shopping, you'll want to get an idea of your bra size. You'll need a tape measure. Either have someone do the measuring for you, or do it yourself. Stand in front of a mirror, wearing nothing on top or only a thin undershirt. Stand tall and breathe normally.

First measure your band size (the number part). Wrap the tape measure around your rib cage right under the bust as shown in the left drawing in Figure 17. Be sure the tape is even, and isn't hiked up in the back. The tape should be snug, but not tight. Once you've done the measurement add 5 to that number. If the result is an odd number, add 1.

Example: The measurement around the chest and under the bust is 26 inches. Adding 5 to 26 equals 31. Since 31 is an odd number add 1. The band size is 32.

Next measure your cup size (the letter part). Measure around your breasts at the fullest part (probably at the nipple level), as shown in the second drawing in Figure 17. Compare this measurement to your band size.

- If the band size is larger than the measurement around your nipples, your cup size is AAA.

- If the band size and the measurement around your nipples are the same, your cup size is AA.

- If the band size is smaller than the measurement, use this guide:

Up to 1" = A	Up to 4" = D
Up to 2" = B	Up to 5" = DD
Up to 3" = C	Up to 6" = E

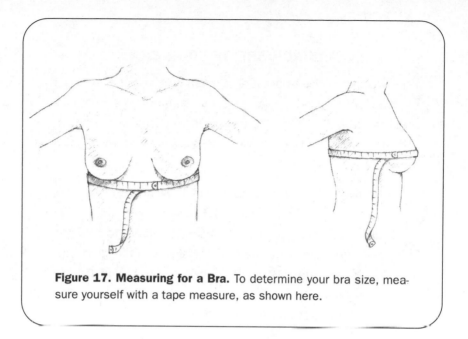

Figure 17. Measuring for a Bra. To determine your bra size, measure yourself with a tape measure, as shown here.

Don't rely on measurements alone, though. Always try a bra on and make sure it fits comfortably before you buy it.

Finding the Right Bra

Finding the right bra isn't always easy. (This is where a fitter can be helpful.) Try different sizes, styles, and brands before you make your choice.

If your breasts spill out on the sides or top, try a bra with a larger cup size. If the cup wrinkles or puckers, the bra is too big. Try a smaller cup size or different style. Look for a bra with adjustable straps. They allow you to adjust the fit for each breast. The bra should fit snugly, but not tightly. You should be able to slip two fingers under the band in back. The band shouldn't ride up. It should be straight across the back. To check the fit, clap your hands over your head. If the bra moves up, it doesn't fit properly.

TAKING CARE OF YOUR BRA

No, you don't have to put it on a leash and take it for a walk! Without proper care, though, your bra can turn into a limp, useless rag. Always read (and follow) any instructions for the care of the bra. In general, following these rules should keep your bras in shape.

- **Washing:** Don't use chlorine bleach. It weakens the elastic in the bra. Washing by hand in lukewarm water is best. For machine washing, choose the coolest setting. To help prevent stretching during machine washing, use a lingerie bag. This fine-mesh or loose-weave bag protects your delicate washables. (Bras go in the bag and the bag goes in the machine along with the rest of the wash.)

- **Drying:** Don't put cotton bras, underwire bras, or bras with trimmings into the dryer. The tumbling and heat (even on low) can cause shrinkage, damage to wires, or fraying. Some types of plain nylon bras can be put in the dryer on the low heat setting. Always check labels to be sure.

- **Give your bra a break:** You shouldn't wear the same bra more than two days in a row. Otherwise, the elastic will wear out more quickly.

In the front, the center of the bra should lie flat against the breastbone. If it lifts off the breastbone, try a larger band size. Also, try a larger band size if the straps pinch your shoulders or if underwires cut into you.

When you find one you like, try it on in another size. Try one that is the next *smallest* band size *and* the next *largest* cup size. For example, if the bra you've found is a 36B, try the same bra in a 34C. Choose the more comfortable one.

Types and Styles

Breasts come in all shapes and sizes. (See Figure 18.) So do bras. *Padded bras* and *falsies,* or inserts, make your breasts appear larger. The padded bra has a pad of cotton or foam rubber inside the cup. Falsies are breast-shaped inserts that are worn inside the cup of a bra.

Push-up bras are often padded. They also push your breasts together, so they look larger. *Underwire* bras have a flexible wire sewn into the lower edge and sides of the cup for support. They

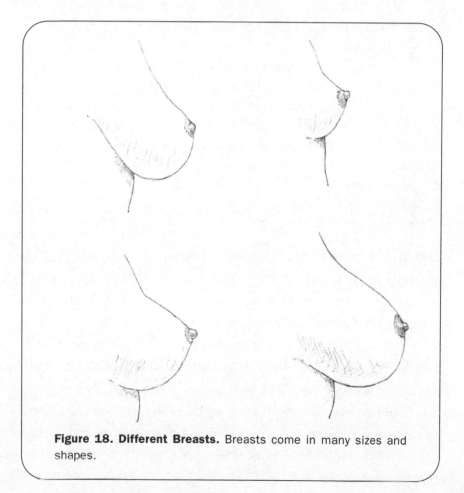

Figure 18. Different Breasts. Breasts come in many sizes and shapes.

SPORTS BRAS

If you're into sports, you need a good sports bra. The good ones are made of material that draws perspiration away from the breasts. This helps keep you cool.

Sports bras restrict breast movement in one of two ways. Compression-type bras press the breasts against the chest wall. They work well for small to medium-size breasts. For larger breasts, sports bras with molded cups work better. The molded cups are also a good choice for extra protection (playing basketball or soccer, for example). Make sure your sports bra has at least 25 percent Lycra or some other material that restricts side-to-side movement.

Forget bras with seams across the nipples. The seams can cause pain and irritation (a condition known as "jogger's nipple"). Check that the bra doesn't chafe around the underarm, rib cage, or across the back. Bra fasteners should be covered, so metal won't push into the skin. Make sure the straps don't dig into the shoulders. Jump up and down and jog in place to check the fit before you buy.

also lift the breasts for a fuller look. They come with full or demi (partial) cups. The demi cups may not provide enough support for large breasts. The full-cup style gives a smooth look under snug tops and helps control jiggling.

Soft-cup bras don't have underwires. They are usually more comfortable to wear. They may not control jiggling as well, though. There are also bras with seams in the cup. Two or more pieces of material have been sewn together to form the cup. These bras lift the breasts and give them a more pleasing shape, but seamless bras look better under knit tops.

FEELINGS ABOUT DEVELOPING BREASTS

Girls are often really excited about their breasts developing. One girl told us:

> I was so happy when my breasts started growing. First, my nipples got bigger. Then my breasts started sticking out. I was so proud. I felt real grown up. I was always showing them off to my mom and my little sister.
>
> —SHARON, AGE 13

Several women remembered feeling embarrassed about their breasts. A twenty-two-year-old told us:

> I used to wrap one of those bandages—the kind you put on a sprained ankle—around my chest to make me flat. I kept my coat on as much as I could and I wore baggy clothes all the time. Now that I'm older, I can laugh about it, but back then it wasn't funny at all.
>
> —NADINE, AGE 22

Women who developed early weren't the only ones who felt embarrassed. Women who were late to develop often felt embarrassed, too. One woman, now in her thirties, told us:

> I didn't start to develop until after my sixteenth birthday. Everyone, and I mean everyone, had breasts but me. They were all in their bras, and there I was in my undershirt. I flunked gym in high school because I wouldn't take a shower. I was too embarrassed about my flat chest. Finally, my mom bought me a padded bra. My breasts did eventually start to

develop, but I really felt bad about myself for a lot of years before they did.

—CECILIA, AGE 33

Another woman told us:

I didn't start developing until I was seventeen. I thought there was something horribly wrong. Maybe I was really a man instead of a woman. Oh, and the teasing I had to endure! The boys used to call me "ironing board" because my chest was so flat.

—MARGARET, AGE 56

Even some girls who developed at the same time as most other girls said they felt embarrassed. As one girl put it:

I started to develop just about the same time as everyone else. I was glad that I was getting tits, but I was embarrassed, especially at school.

—KIM, AGE 16

UNWANTED ATTENTION AND SEXUAL HARASSMENT

Our families, our friends, or kids at school may tease us about developing breasts. Even strangers may make comments about our changing bodies. Boys or men may whistle or make sexual remarks. One girl liked this kind of attention:

---

harassment (huh-RASS-ment)

If I'm walking down the street and some guy says, "Hey, there!" or whistles or something, I feel pretty good, like he's saying, "Oh, you look good," especially if I'm with a girl-friend or a bunch of girls.

—MYRA, AGE 16

Most girls don't like this kind of attention. One girl said:

I hate when boys stare at my breasts or whistle or yell stuff at me. It makes me feel like a piece of meat. It makes me feel self-conscious and dumb. I mean, what can you do? Yell back at them? How would they like it if girls went down the street and stared at their crotches and yelled stuff like, "Hey, that's a really big penis you got there!" Boys do that. They say stuff like, "Hey, that's a great set of jugs!" I don't like it.

—RENEE, AGE 14

How you handle this kind of unwanted attention depends on the situation. If it comes from strangers—for example, some guys driving by in a car—it's probably best to ignore it. There are too many crazies in the world. You don't want to get into a shouting match on the street with some nut.

In other situations, you may be able to handle things differently. Suppose you walk by a construction site or store on your way to school each day. There's a group of guys who work or hang out there. Each day, as you walk by, they make noises, gestures, or sexual remarks. In this kind of situation, you or your parents could contact the store owner or head of the company. Tell them about the problem and point out that they're responsible for stopping it.

ERICA'S STORY

This following is from Erica's website for victims of sexual harassment: (http://erosen.tripod.com/shhelp/index.html):

If you have been harassed by other students, you may have been made to feel it's just a case of "boys will be boys." Like many victims, you may simply accept it as something you just have to deal with. But harassment at a young age can have very damaging effects.

I know about the problems that can develop when you face something like this. As a victim of harassment, I have searched for a way to find support from other victims. I called many groups—from rape [counseling] centers to organizations that educate about harassment. I was told that I could join a support group for victims of sexual assault.

The counselor said I was facing issues similar to those of a woman who has been raped [forced to have sex—see page 232]. I was afraid those who had been physically hurt would resent me. Perhaps they would feel my problems were not as bad as theirs. The counselor assured me they would be supportive.

All the group members had the same story. One day it, the rape, happened. Their lives changed. They were filled with pain and anger at the person who had done this to them. They wondered when they would feel like themselves again.

Many said things I had always felt. The emotions were similar. But I didn't hear some of the key things that were worst for me. I felt that I never got a chance to develop my personality before the harassment began. I didn't have a "me" to go back to being. This wasn't just some horrible thing that happened one day. I had to go through it every single

Unwanted attention from strangers is annoying. It can be more than annoying when it comes from people you know and happens at school or in your neighborhood. If this happens often, your school or neighborhood can change into a place of daily pain. When unwanted attention goes this far, it becomes *sexual* day for years. Every day I was expected to sit in a classroom with those who harassed me. I had to work with them on school projects. I had to live in the neighborhood with them. I had to live with girls telling me I was a slut based on how guys talked to me. It didn't matter that I had never been sexually active in my life.

What happened to me happened in front of adults. A rape victim could have gone to them for help. But, in my case, it was dismissed as adolescent behavior and nothing was said. Teachers would only ask if some problem at home was the cause of my falling grades. Once a female dance teacher told me I needed a sports bra because all the guys were staring at me.

I know there must be thousands of victims. But I don't think they realize what they have gone through. I didn't. Because my teachers didn't help me, I accepted it. I hid the pain and anger away inside me. Not until it finally exploded did I realize how much It had affected me.

The harassment didn't only affect me. It also affected the young girls who saw it. It sent the message that it is acceptable to be treated like a sex object and humiliated because something about one's body is beautiful.

I know the boys who harassed me thought it was okay to treat women like that. One of them attends the same university as I do. Last year, he called me at all hours of the night. He wanted me to come meet him so we could "have a good time." Later he raped a girl who lived in his dorm.

I made a website for those who have faced the "boys will be boys" attitude.

harassment. One girl's experience with this kind of harassment is recounted in "Erica's Story."

No one has the right to make sexual comments, gestures, or advances to you if you don't want them to, not your classmates or neighbors, not your teachers, nor any other adults. Any type of unwelcome behavior of a sexual nature can be considered sexual harassment.

Sexual harassment takes many forms—verbal, written, or physical. It can include joking, teasing, requests for sexual favors, comments about your body, remarks or questions about past or present sexual activities, "dirty" jokes or stories, spreading sexual rumors, or threats of sexual violence. It might also be in the form of sexual graffiti, notes or pictures or suggestive gestures, looks, or leers. Sometimes sexual harassment involves physical contact, including touching or grabbing.

Often, sexual harassment takes place at school. In one large survey, eight out of ten teens said they'd been sexually harassed at school. Both males and females can be victims and both can be harassers. In the same survey, nearly seven out of ten males and five out of ten females admitted to harassing other students. Teachers and other adults can be the harassers, but harassment by students is much more common. When it's students harassing other students, it's called "peer sexual harassment."

Dealing with Peer Sexual Harassment

Too often, we are told to "just ignore it." Maybe this advice puts an end to harassment sometimes. In most cases, though, sexual harassment doesn't stop unless or until someone confronts the harasser and tells him or her to stop.

There are a number of things you can do if you're harassed at school. What you do depends on what happens, how often it happens, and how serious it is. Here are some suggestions:

- Tell the harasser to stop.

- Write the harasser a letter. (You could mail the letter, deliver it yourself, or get another kid or an adult to deliver it.)

- Get a parent, teacher, or school counselor to help you. (The harasser may be more likely to listen to an adult.)

- Report the problem to your principal. Ask to see a copy of your school's sexual harassment policy.

If nothing else works, the last suggestion on the list should get you some action. School districts have been sued successfully for large amounts of money for failing to respond to student complaints. These cases involved repeated incidents of peer sexual harassment when the problem was serious enough to affect the student's education. The lawsuits were brought under Title IX of the Federal Education Act, which prohibits sex discrimination in the public schools. Your school district will have a Title IX Coordinator. Ask to speak to that person. (For more information, see the Resource Section at the back of the book.) In view of these lawsuits, it's likely that your complaint will be taken seriously by school officials.

We hope you will find a way to stop any sexual harassment that may come your way. Puberty is a special time. It is a time to feel proud of your developing sexuality. Nobody should be allowed to interfere with these good feelings.

3.
PUBIC HAIR AND OTHER CHANGES "DOWN THERE"

Women from earlier generations never talked about their sex organs. If forced to mention "such things," they said "private parts" or "down there." But you know that *vulva* is the name for the sex organs on the outside of your body.

In Chapter 1, you learned the names of some parts of the vulva—the mons, the clitoris, the inner and outer lips. In this chapter, we'll take you on a guided tour of your own body. You'll learn more about the different parts of the vulva and how they change as you go through puberty.

One change in the vulva is the growth of *pubic hair*. In this chapter, you'll learn about the five stages of pubic hair growth. For most girls, pubic hair or breast development is the first sign of puberty, so we'll also talk about ages and stages and the start of puberty in this chapter.

During puberty, the vulva becomes very sensitive to sexual thoughts and feelings. At the end of this chapter, you'll find a discussion of this change in the vulva.

PUBIC HAIR

In adult women, curly *pubic hair* covers the mons in a triangle pattern. During puberty, the first pubic hairs appear. Your first hairs may not be very dark. As puberty continues, they get darker. In the end, your pubic hair probably will be as dark or darker than the hair on your head, or it may be a different color entirely. Pubic hair comes in all colors—blond, brown, black, and red.

Some women have lots of pubic hair. Others have less. How much you have will depend on your own body chemistry and your family background. Ethnic or racial background may play a role. For example, some experts say Asians tend to have less pubic hair than women from other backgrounds. (The experts don't, however, say just who they mean by "Asians.")

Feelings About Pubic Hair

For some girls, pubic hair is the first sign of puberty. Some girls we talked to were excited about growing pubic hair. Others weren't 100 percent happy. Many girls said they were both excited and, at times, scared or uncertain. Here's what girls we talked with had to say:

> One day I was taking a bath. I noticed three little curly hairs growing down there. I started yelling for my mom to come and see. I felt real grown up.
>
> —JOCELYN, AGE 9

NO PLUCKING, PLEASE!

I saw these curly, black hairs. I didn't know what they were, so I got the tweezers and pulled them out. Pretty soon, they grew back. Then there were more and more of them. So I figured it must be okay.

—KATE, AGE 9

Several girls said they plucked their first pubic hairs. This won't get rid of your pubic hairs. They'll just grow back. And, ouch! Plucking pubic hairs hurts!

I just wasn't ready. I remember when I first saw that my pubic hairs were growing. I thought, oh, no, I don't want this to start happening to me yet. Then I got breasts. It was like I suddenly started having this grown-up body, but I still felt like a kid inside.

—MEGAN, AGE 13

I was afraid I was going to have to be all grown up and wear high heels all the time instead of being a tomboy and climbing trees, but, really, it turned out that I did just the same things I always did.

—JANELLE, AGE 15

You may feel good or bad (or a bit of both) about the changes happening in your body. In any case, it helps to have someone you can talk to about your feelings. Reading this book with someone might be a good way for you to start talking about these changes.

FIVE STAGES OF PUBIC HAIR GROWTH

Doctors divide pubic hair growth into five stages. These stages are shown in Figure 19. Read about the different stages in the next pages. Then compare your body to the drawings in Figure 19. Which stage best matches your pubic hair growth?

By the way, breast and pubic hair stages don't always match. You may be in one stage of breast development and in a different stage of pubic hair growth. For example, you might be in Stage 2 of breast development and Stage 1 of pubic hair growth (or vice versa). So, don't worry if your breast and pubic hair stages don't match. It's perfectly normal! When breast and pubic hair stages don't match, there's usually not a big difference between the two. This isn't always the case, though. Sometimes one type of development is quite a bit slower than the other. For example, sometimes a girl is in Stage 4 of breast development before she grows her first pubic hair. This, too, is perfectly normal.

Stage 1: Childhood

This is the childhood, or prepuberty, stage. There is no pubic hair. You may have some hair on the vulva in this stage. If so, it's the light, downy type of hair that grows on the belly and other places. This childhood hair is short, fine, soft, and has little color. It is not pubic hair.

Stage 2: First Pubic Hairs Appear

This stage starts when the first pubic hairs appear. The first hairs are straight or a bit curly. They have some color, but not much. They are coarser and longer than the childhood hairs seen in Stage 1. These first hairs usually grow on the edges of the outer lips.

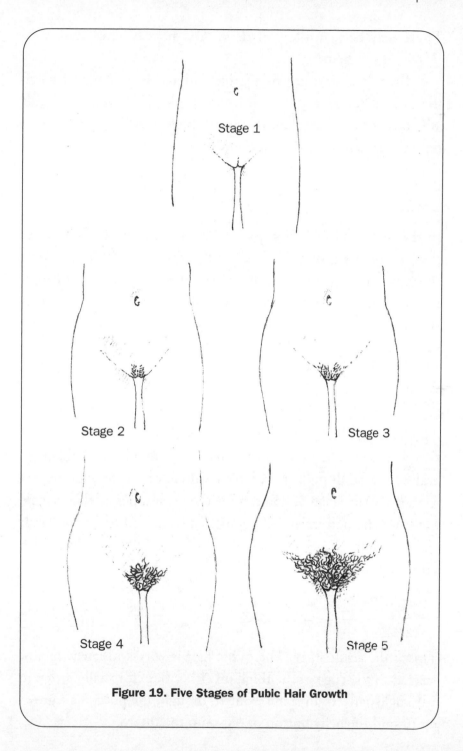

Figure 19. Five Stages of Pubic Hair Growth

There may be just a few of them. You may have to look very closely to see them.

Most girls start growing pubic hair and begin Stage 2 when they are eight and a half to eleven years old. However, some girls are younger or older than this when they start Stage 2. Stage 2 typically lasts nine to sixteen months.

Stage 3: Growth Extends to Mons

In this stage, pubic hair grows on the mons as well as the outer lips. The hairs grow mostly on the center of the mons, above the lips. There are more pubic hairs than in Stage 2, but still not very many. The hairs are also darker and curlier in this stage. Stage 3 may last for a matter of months or for two years or more.

Stage 4: Growth Continues

There is a good deal more pubic hair than there was in Stage 3. It covers more of the mons. The pubic hairs are now as dark, curly, and wiry as adult pubic hair, but they do not cover as wide an area as they will in Stage 5. You can see the beginnings of the triangle pattern. The pattern is not yet as clear as it will be in the adult stage. Usually Stage 4 lasts anywhere from eight months to two years or more.

Stage 5: Adult

This is the adult stage. The pubic hair is wiry and curly. It now reaches to the edge of the thigh on either side. It usually grows in a triangle pattern. In some women, though, the pubic hair grows up toward the belly button or out onto the thighs.

Pubic Hair Stages and Your First Period

Most girls have their first period when they are in Pubic Hair Stage 3 or 4. There are also some who don't get their first period until Stage 5. A few girls start their periods while they are still in Pubic Hair Stage 2, though this is rare.

If you have your period or any bleeding before you develop either breasts or pubic hair, you need to see a doctor and get it checked out.

STARTING PUBERTY: AGES AND STAGES

Pubic hair may be the first outward sign that a girl is starting puberty. In fact, pubic hairs or breast buds (or both) are the first sign of puberty for most girls. When a girl reaches Stage 2 of either pubic hair growth or breast development, she officially starts puberty.

But remember: Different girls start puberty at different ages. We each have our own personal timetable of development.

Take the girls in Figure 20, for example. Both girls are completely healthy and normal in every way. The girl on the right is only ten years old. She has already started puberty. In fact, she's already in Stage 3 of breast development and Stage 3 of pubic hair growth. The girl on the left is almost twelve years old. She hasn't begun to develop. She hasn't started puberty yet.

These girls have different timetables and are at different stages of development, but both girls are developing normally, at the right age and time for their own bodies.

Starting Early/Starting Late—Why?

Why do some girls start early, at a young age, and others not until they're older? We don't know the complete answer to this ques-

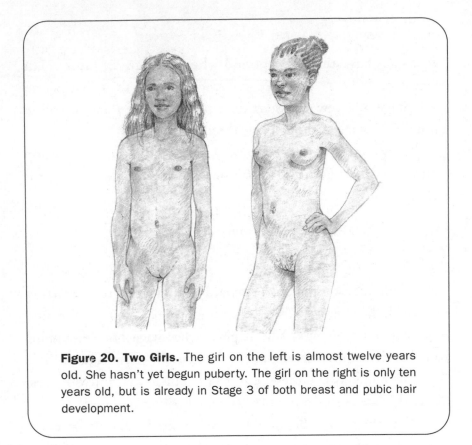

Figure 20. Two Girls. The girl on the left is almost twelve years old. She hasn't yet begun puberty. The girl on the right is only ten years old, but is already in Stage 3 of both breast and pubic hair development.

tion. Some of what we do know is pretty surprising. For example, *where* you live may affect *when* you start puberty. Girls who live high in the mountains begin to develop later than girls who live near sea level. Diet and nutrition can also affect the age at which puberty starts. Girls who are undernourished tend to develop later than girls who have proper diets. On the other hand, girls who are overweight tend to develop earlier than girls of normal weight.

Family Background

Your family background has a lot to do with when you start to develop. Girls tend to take after their female relatives. For example, if the women in your family started puberty at an early age, chances are, you will, too. If you come from a family of late starters, you probably won't start puberty until you're older.

This is not a hard-and-fast rule. You may differ from your family. For instance, a girl whose female relatives were late starters could begin puberty at the average age or even earlier. Also, your female relatives may not have a common pattern. They may be a mix of average, early, and late starters. But females from the same family are often alike in this way. So it's worth asking your relatives when they started to develop.

Puberty Is Starting Earlier Today

Are most of your female relatives more than ten years older than you? If so, you may start puberty at an earlier age than they did. Girls today seem to be developing breasts and pubic hair earlier than they did ten or twenty years ago.

In the past, on average, breast and pubic hair development started around eleven or twelve. However, in 1997, a new study showed girls developing at younger ages. This study involved over 17,000 white and African-American girls, ages three through twelve. On the average, African-American girls started puberty between eight and nine years of age. On the average, white girls started later, at around ten years of age.

There were also many girls in the study who developed at even younger ages. Twenty-seven percent of the seven-year-old African-American girls had started to develop either breasts or pubic hair or both. About 7 percent of the seven-year-old white girls had begun either breast development or pubic hair growth or both. (*Twenty-seven percent* means twenty seven out of every one hundred. *Seven percent* means seven out of every one hundred.)

Racial and Ethnic Background

Different racial and ethnic groups may have different average ages for starting puberty. In our country, we have girls from many different racial and ethnic groups. Unfortunately, we don't have up-to-date studies on all these different groups. The study mentioned above, which compares African-American and white girls, is one of the few such studies. It showed, on the average, African-American girls begin to develop a year or so earlier than white girls. We don't completely understand why these differences exist. Nor do we know much about other racial or ethnic groups. But our best guess is that, on average, girls from other racial and ethnic groups probably start puberty within a few months of white girls.

Remember, though, not everyone is average. There are some girls who develop breasts and pubic hair long before, or long after, the average girl in their group. Also, there are plenty of white girls who develop *before* some of their African-American classmates. As difficult as it is to be different, you have to remember there is no "right" age for everyone. Your body is developing at the age that's right for you.

Am I Normal?

Seems like everyone asks this question at some point during puberty. The answer is almost always "yes," but sometimes a medical problem can delay puberty or cause it to start too early. It's not always easy to know what's "too early" or "too late," so, in the next pages, we'll give some guidelines on when you should see a doctor. Doctors can treat these kinds of problems.

Sometimes a girl's classmates have all started puberty, but she hasn't shown any signs at all. This usually means the girl is just a late starter. Every once in a while, though, a girl may have a medical problem that keeps her from starting puberty. As a general rule, girls who haven't developed any signs of puberty by their thirteenth or fourteenth birthday should see a doctor. In other words, a girl who is still in Breast Stage 1 *and* in Pubic Hair Stage 1 by her fourteenth birthday should be checked by a doctor. Because they usually develop earlier, an African-American girl should use her thirteenth birthday as the guide.

Girls who are early starters often worry just as much as the late starters. In most cases, though, being an early starter doesn't mean there's anything wrong with you. It just means that you are developing sooner than other girls. Once in a while, though, being an early starter can be a sign of a medical problem. African-American girls who develop pubic hair or breasts before the age of six should see a doctor. Other girls should see a doctor if they begin developing before the age of seven.

Of course, you don't have to always follow these guidelines. If you feel that something isn't right with the way your body is developing, see your doctor no matter what age you are. If it turns out that you do have a medical problem, you'll have caught it that much earlier. If you don't have a problem, you'll feel better knowing there's nothing wrong.

YOUR VULVA—A GUIDED TOUR

Now, back to the changes in your vulva. Figure 21 shows the vulva in a girl who has finished going through puberty. If you haven't yet started or are just beginning puberty, your vulva will not be the same as that of a fully developed girl. During childhood the outer lips are smooth and hairless, and the inner lips are not very noticeable. The urinary and vaginal openings are tiny and hard to see. During puberty, pubic hair begins to grow on the mons and outer lips. The inner lips become fleshy. The clitoris is larger. The urinary and vaginal openings are also larger and easier to see than they are in childhood. The *hymen,* a thin piece of tissue just inside the vaginal opening, is also more noticeable. (We'll talk more about the hymen as we continue our tour.)

In the mature girl shown in Figure 21 the pubic hair has reached Stage 5. The inner and outer lips are quite plump. The clitoris, urinary opening, and vaginal opening are adult-size.

The girl at the top of Figure 21 is using a mirror to look at her vulva. With a mirror, it's easy to see the different parts of the vulva. You can learn about these organs by comparing your own body to this drawing. You probably won't look *exactly* like this drawing. You may not be as mature as this girl. Each person's body is a little bit different, just as each person's face is. Still, you can compare this drawing to your own body and try to find the parts of your vulva. With a little practice, the features of your vulva will become as plain as the nose on your face.

Some girls think it's great to use a mirror to learn about their body. As one girl in our class said:

> Oh, I've looked at myself there lots of times. My mom got a mirror and told me how to look at myself and showed me pictures so I'd know what I'll look like when I grow up. She taught me the names of everything and all that stuff.
>
> —CARLA, AGE 10

Some girls don't feel as comfortable about touching or looking at their genitals. Another girl said:

> I thought it sounded kind of weird, taking a mirror and looking at myself down there, but I was kind of curious. So I

---

hymen (HI-mun)

locked my bedroom door and took a good look. I'm glad I did. It made me feel like I know more about myself, like it wasn't such a big mystery.

—RUBY, AGE 12

Still another girl said:

Ugh, that's disgusting. I'd never do that. It's yucky down there.

—CYNTHIA, AGE 11

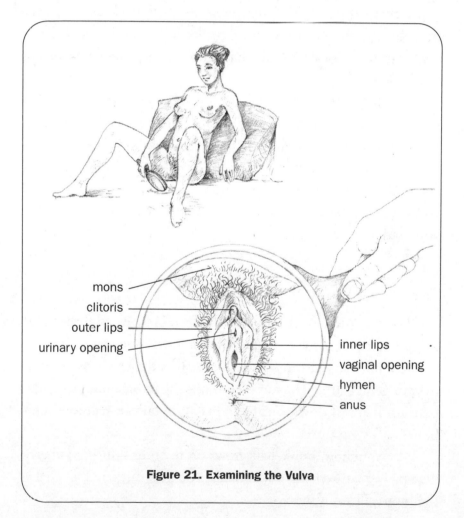

Figure 21. Examining the Vulva

Some girls are taught that their genitals are "dirty" or that it is wrong to look at or touch them. Even if no one has actually said this, you may still feel uneasy about looking at your genitals. People don't talk about genital organs very much. And, as we all know, if something is too terrible to talk about, then it must be really terrible!

But there is nothing terrible or dirty about the vulva. Some people may feel uneasy because it is a sexual part of the body, and they're uncomfortable with anything that has to do with sex. Other people think the genitals are dirty because the openings through which urine and feces leave our bodies are in this area. But our mouths usually have more germs than this area of our bodies.

In the following pages, we'll take a guided tour of the vulva. We'll explain how your genitals change during puberty. If you don't feel okay about touching or looking at your genitals, that's fine. Just read these pages and look at the drawings. We don't want you to do anything you don't feel okay doing. If you'd like to, though, you can use a mirror to look at yourself as you read.

The Mons

We'll start our tour at the top of the vulva. Here we find the *mons*. It is a pad of fat tissue over the pubic bone. If you stand sideways before a mirror, you can see the mons. It is the small rise of flesh in your genital area. The mons cushions the pubic bones which lie beneath it. Press down on the mons and you can feel the pubic bones.

As you know, pubic hair grows on the mons during puberty. The pad of fat over the pubic bones also gets thicker. This makes the mons stick out more.

THERE'S ANOTHER NAME FOR IT

Mons is a Latin word meaning "little hill or mound." The mons also has a longer name: *mons veneris. Veneris* is another Latin word. It refers to Venus, the goddess of love. So the longer name means "mound of Venus" or "mound of love."

The mons is also called the *mons pubis* because it protects the pubic bones. Another name from the same root is *pubes. Pubes* refers to either pubic hair or the pubic bones.

The inner and outer lips are also called the *vaginal lips*, or *labia. Labia* is the Latin word for lips. *Majora* is another Latin word. It means "first in importance or size." The outer lips come before the inner lips and are usually larger. That's why the medical name for the outer lips is *labia majora*. The medical name for the inner lips is *labia minora. Minora* comes from the same Latin root as our word minor.

The Outer Lips

The lower part of the mons divides into two folds of skin. These are the *outer lips*. They are rather flat and smooth before puberty. During puberty, fat tissue makes them thicker. In old age, the lips may lose fat and become flat and smooth again.

In children, the outer lips usually don't touch. But when the lips get fatter during puberty, they often begin to touch. In grown women, the lips usually touch. After childbirth or in old age, the lips may separate again.

---

veneris (VEN-air-iss)
pubis (PEW-bis)
pubes (PEW-beez)
labia (LAY-bee-uh)
majora (muh-JOR-uh)
minora (mi-NOR-uh)

The undersides of the lips are hairless. In children, the undersides are also smooth. During puberty, you may notice small bumps dotting the skin on the undersides of the lips. These are oil glands. They make a small amount of oil, which keeps the area moist and protects against irritation. There are also special sweat glands in the outer lips. These glands mature at puberty, and may cause a change in your body odor. (For more information, see pages 113–116.)

During childhood, this area may be light pink to red to brownish-black in color. It depends on your skin tone. The color is apt to change during puberty.

The Inner Lips

If you separate the outer lips, you will see two *inner lips*. During childhood, the inner lips are small. During puberty, they grow and become more noticeable. Like the outer lips, they protect the area between them. They tend to change color and get more wrinkly during puberty.

Figure 22 shows the inner lips in different women. In most women, the inner lips are smaller than the outer lips, but in some women the inner lips stick out further than the outer lips. The two inner lips are usually about the same size. Sometimes, though, one is larger than the other.

The inner lips are hairless in both girls and grown women. They usually become more moist as we go through puberty. They too have oil glands that begin making more oil during puberty.

The Clitoris

If you follow the inner lips upward toward the mons, you will see that they come together. In the area where they meet lies the tip of

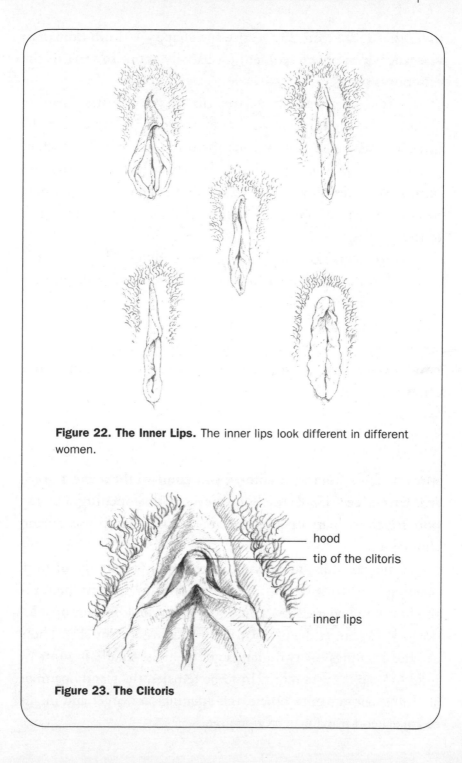

Figure 22. The Inner Lips. The inner lips look different in different women.

hood

tip of the clitoris

inner lips

Figure 23. The Clitoris

the *clitoris*. (See Figure 23.) Its size and shape vary from woman to woman, but in grown women, it's usually about the size of the eraser on a pencil.

A fold of tissue above the tip of the clitoris forms a "hood." The hood may cover some or all of the tip of the clitoris. You may have to pull back the hood to see it. Even then, you will see only its tip. The rest of the clitoris is under the skin. If you press down on the skin above the clitoris, you may be able to feel a rubbery cord under the skin. This is the shaft of the clitoris.

The clitoris has many, many nerve endings. They make the clitoris and the area around it very sensitive to direct or indirect touch or pressure. Touching this area of the body can give us excited, tingly kinds of feelings. In fact, the clitoris is an organ of sexual pleasure for females. At the end of this chapter, we'll talk more about sexual pleasure. For now, though, let's continue our tour of the vulva.

The Urinary Opening

Moving down from your clitoris, you come to the *urinary opening*. Urine (pee) leaves the body through this opening. During puberty, the urinary opening becomes larger than it was during childhood.

It may be difficult for you to see exactly where the urinary opening is. Moving down from the clitoris in a straight line, it is the first dimpled area you come to. It may look like an upside-down *V*. On both sides of the urinary opening are tiny slits. These are the openings for two glands. They make small amounts of fluid to keep the area moist. In some females, the gland openings are too small to see. In others, the openings are larger and might be mistaken for the urinary opening.

The Vaginal Opening

Once you find the urinary opening, it's easy to find the *vaginal opening*. Just move down from the urinary opening in a straight line and you'll come to the vaginal opening. (Remember, the vagina itself is tucked up inside the body.)

In young girls, the opening to the vagina is not very big. During puberty, the vagina starts to grow and the vaginal opening gets bigger. Drawings of the vaginal opening can be very confusing. They often show the vaginal opening as a black hole. It's not.

The vagina is like a balloon. Both the vagina and its opening can expand to many times their size. They can stretch enough for a man's penis to fit in there during sex. When a woman has a baby, they expand even more. This lets the baby pass through the vagina during childbirth. Most of the time, the vagina isn't stretched and its sides lie flat against each other. It's like a balloon that hasn't been blown up yet. Imagine what you'd see if you looked into the opening in the neck of a collapsed balloon. You wouldn't see a black hole. You'd see the inside surfaces of the balloon pressed up against each other. The same is true of the vagina. If you look into the vaginal opening, you don't see a black hole. You see the inside walls of the vagina pressed up against each other.

If you're using a mirror to look at your own body, check it out. We guarantee you won't see a black hole. However, we won't promise you'll see the inside walls of your vagina. Your hymen may be in the way.

The Hymen

The hymen is also called the "maidenhead" or (in slang) the "cherry." It is a thin piece of tissue just inside the vaginal opening. Hymens come in many sizes and shapes. Some hymens are just a

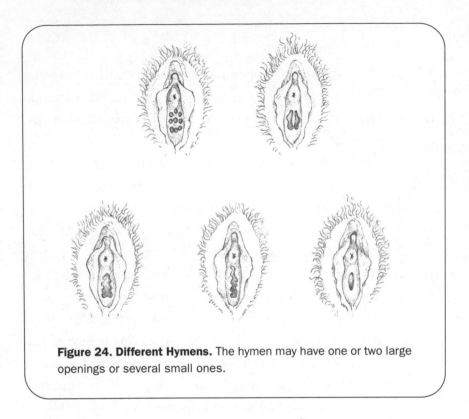

Figure 24. Different Hymens. The hymen may have one or two large openings or several small ones.

rim of tissue ringing the vaginal opening. Other hymens stretch all or part way across the vaginal opening and have one or more openings. (These openings allow the menstrual flow to leave the body when a girl has her period.) Figure 24 shows some different types of hymens.

Even with a mirror, you may not be able to identify your hymen. Before puberty, the hymen is very thin. If you haven't started puberty, you may have difficulty seeing it. During puberty, the hymen gets thicker. It may become ruffled and develop folds. These changes make the hymen easier to see, but you may have trouble telling the folds of a ruffly hymen from the folds of the vaginal walls. In females who have had sex, the hymen usually doesn't look like any of the ones shown in Figure 24. When a female has sex for the first time, the erect penis

CAN A DOCTOR TELL?

If a doctor examines your hymen can he or she tell if you've had sexual intercourse?

Girls ask this question for different reasons. Some are just curious. Some have had sexual intercourse and are worried about the doctor finding out about it. Others have been victims of sexual abuse or rape (forced intercourse), and they want to know if the condition of their hymen can be used as evidence.

A doctor can't tell for certain whether or not a girl has had sex from the condition of her hymen. A hymen that doesn't appear to be stretched or torn can *suggest* that a girl hasn't had sex, but can't prove it. The reason: some girls have sex many times without stretching or tearing their hymens. And the reverse applies, too. Although a hymen that appears to have been stretched or torn can *suggest* that a girl has had sex, it doesn't prove it. Some girls have hymens that appear stretched or torn even though they haven't been and the girls have never had sex. In cases of sexual abuse, a stretched or torn hymen could be used, along with other evidence, to support the charge of abuse. But the condition of the hymen alone usually isn't proof of sexual activity.

entering the vagina usually causes some stretching or even tearing of the hymen. (This may cause a small amount of bleeding and some discomfort or pain, though this usually isn't severe or long-lasting.) In females who've begun having sex, the hymen may be nothing more than a few tags of tissue or an irregular fringe of tissue.

Sexual intercourse is the most common way of stretching or tearing the hymen, but accidents or injuries can stretch or tear the hymen, too. However, injuries that penetrate the vagina and tear the hymen are very rare. Perhaps you've heard that activities like horseback riding, gymnastics, or other such sports can tear or stretch the hymen. But recent studies show that this is not the case.

The Anus

Moving down from the vaginal opening, you come to the *anus*. Feces leave the body through this opening. The skin around the anus may get a little darker during puberty. Pubic hair may also start to grow here. The anus isn't really part of the vulva, though. We mention it only because it's in the same area of your body.

This completes the tour of the vulva. During puberty, the vulva may become very sensitive to sexual thoughts and feelings. The clitoris and the area around it are especially sensitive. This area of the body can be the source of strong sexual sensations. So, before leaving this chapter, we want to talk about *masturbation* and the female sexual response.

MASTURBATION

Touching, rubbing, or otherwise stimulating the genital organs for sexual pleasure is called *masturbating*. Females most commonly masturbate by touching, rubbing, or stroking the clitoris or other parts of the vulva.

Not everyone masturbates. Most of us do, though. People of all ages and both sexes masturbate. (Males masturbate by rubbing, touching, or stroking their penises.) Some of us start masturbating when we're children and continue to do so all our lives. Some of us start during puberty. Some of us don't start until we are

---

masturbation (mass-tur-BAY-shun)
masturbating (MASS-tur-bate-ing)

older. Some of us never masturbate. It's normal if you do it and normal if you don't.

You may have heard all sorts of strange stories about masturbation. People used to think that masturbation would make you insane or blind or turn you into a moron. These stories aren't true. (If they were, there would be an awful lot of insane, blind morons around!) You may have heard that masturbation will make you enjoy sex with another person less. Also not true. Masturbating is a way of practicing for your adult sex life. Learning how to give yourself pleasure can be the first step in learning how to have sexual pleasure with someone else some day.

Can masturbating "too much" hurt a person? The answer is no. Nothing bad will happen to your body regardless of how much you masturbate. Masturbation is not physically harmful in any way. (Your genitals might get a little sore if you are rubbing them a whole lot.)

Some people masturbate every day. Some masturbate many times in one day. Others only rarely masturbate, and still others never do. Some people like to imagine things that excite them when they are masturbating. Imagining or pretending that something is happening is called *fantasizing*. We fantasize about all sorts of things. Almost everyone has fantasies about sex. These fantasies can help us to better know our sexual self. So our advice is: relax and enjoy them.

Having fantasies about sex and masturbating are against some people's religious or moral beliefs, however. Personally, we think masturbation is good for you. And most people believe it's morally acceptable, too. But if you believe masturbation is wrong, you can decide not to do it. In any case, you should know that masturbation is *not* physically harmful in any way. In

---

fantasizing (FAN-tuh-size-ing)

fact, most experts agree that masturbation is healthy, normal, and good for you.

Sexual Arousal and Orgasm

Sexual arousal means "being sexually excited, or turned on." When a female is sexually aroused, she may notice an increased feeling of wetness in her genitals. As you'll learn in Chapter 6, the vagina is normally moist. However, when a female becomes sexually excited, her body produces fluids that lubricate the vagina. This causes an increased sensation of wetness in the vulva.

If you continue masturbating long enough, you may have an *orgasm*. (Some other terms for having an orgasm are "climaxing," "coming," and "getting off.") Orgasm is a release of tension and excitement that builds up in the body during sexual arousal. It's a bit difficult to explain exactly what an orgasm feels like. For one thing, an orgasm can vary from one time to the next. Some orgasms are very powerful and strong. Others are less intense. A less intense one might be described as a "lovely shivery feeling." A powerful one might feel like an explosion, a spasm of intense sexual pleasure that begins in the genitals and pulses throughout the body. Most people agree that an orgasm is a *very* good feeling.

You may not have an orgasm every time you masturbate. For one thing, you may stop before you get to the point of orgasm. Also, having an orgasm means learning what arouses your body. It may take a bit of practice. That's why experts say that masturbation is an excellent way of learning how your body reacts and of practicing for your adult sex life.

---

arousal (uh-RAU-zuhl)
orgasm (OR-gaz-um)

THE G-SPOT

Men usually ejaculate when they have an orgasm. (If you recall, ejaculation is the release of a small amount of creamy fluid from the tip of the penis.) Females don't ejaculate in the sense that men do. However, some women report releasing a spurt of fluid at orgasm. Experts are not sure where this fluid comes from. It may be a small amount of urine or fluid from the slit-like openings of the glands near the urinary opening.

Some experts claim there is a specific spot inside the vagina that, like the clitoris, is super sensitive to sexual stimulation. They also claim that stimulating this spot—which they call the G-spot—will cause the release of fluid at orgasm. Other experts do not believe there is a G-spot, although they do agree that there are sensitive areas inside the vagina.

4.

THE PUBERTY GROWTH SPURT

Are the shoes you bought just last month too small? Are your practically brand-new jeans up around your ankles already? If so, you've probably started your puberty growth spurt.

During puberty, we go through a period of extra-fast growth. We put on weight and grow taller at a faster rate than before puberty. We call this period of super-fast growth the *puberty growth spurt*. It begins at different ages for different girls. It is more dramatic in some girls than in others, but all girls do a good deal of growing at this time. This growth spurt usually lasts for a few years. Then the rate of growth slows back down again and eventually stops.

In this chapter, we'll be talking about several different aspects of the puberty growth spurt. Two of these are the height spurt and the weight spurt, but the puberty growth spurt does more than make you taller and heavier. During puberty certain parts of our bodies grow more than others. The result: your face and body may look quite a bit different than they did before puberty. You start to look more adult and less like a kid!

While you are growing and developing in so many different ways, eating properly and exercising are especially important. But many young people don't do either. Their diets don't have the vitamins and minerals they need and they don't get enough exercise. These problems can have a particularly bad effect on a young person's bones. During puberty you build up the bone strength that will last your whole lifetime. If you don't build enough bone mass in these years, it can cause problems later in life so, in this chapter, we'll also talk about proper diet and exercise during your puberty years.

THE HEIGHT SPURT

Before she hits puberty, the average girl is growing at a rate of about two and a half inches per year. Once the height spurt begins, growth speeds up. A girl's rate of growth may nearly double, so she adds almost four inches to her height in a single year. On the average, a girl adds a total of about nine inches to her height during the puberty growth spurt. Of course, everyone is different, so you may grow more or less than this.

The growth spurt usually lasts about three years. By the time you've had your first menstrual period, your growth rate has usually slowed back down. By then, you're growing only one or two inches a year. Most girls reach their full adult height within one to three years after their first periods.

Boys go through a height spurt during puberty, too, but boys typically start their height spurts later than girls. For girls, the growth spurt happens early in puberty. It is one of the first changes. For boys, the growth spurt is not an early change. It happens later in puberty. On the average, boys' growth spurts happen about two years later than girls' growth spurts. This is why eleven- and twelve-year-old girls are often taller than the boys their age. A couple of years later, the boys start their growth spurt. Then the boys usually catch up to the girls and eventually pass them in height. Of course, some girls—the ones who are on the tall side—will always be taller than many of the boys. But often an eleven- or twelve-year-old girl who is taller than the boys her age will find the boys have caught up by age thirteen or fourteen.

How Tall Will I Be?

We can't tell for sure how tall you'll be, but we can give you a couple of clues.

Your height *before* your growth spurt is one clue. If you are short as a child, it's likely you'll be short as an adult. Likewise, tall children tend to become tall adults. But this is *definitely* not a hard-and-fast rule. For example, many girls told us they were among the shortest in their class before puberty. Then their height spurt started and they ended up being among the tallest girls in their class.

You can get a better idea of your adult height by following the steps below. First, though, you need to know how tall your mom and dad are. (For this exercise, guardians, foster, and adoptive parents won't do. You need to know your birth parents' heights.)

1. Subtract 5 inches from your dad's height.

2. Add your mom's height to the result you got in Step 1.

3. Divide the result you got in Step 2 by 2. The result is your estimated adult height.

Example: Harmony's father is 5 feet, 11 inches tall and her mother is 5 feet, 4 inches tall. First we subtract 5 inches from her father's height. The result is 5 feet, 6 inches. Now add her mother's height (5 feet, 4 inches). The result is 10 feet, 10 inches. Now we divide the result by 2. The result is 5 feet, 5 inches. This is Harmony's estimated adult height. In other words, she should wind up one inch taller than her mother.

Probably your parents are not the same height as Harmony's parents. So you will have to do the math for yourself with the correct heights for your own parents. Remember, though, the result you get in Step 3 is only an estimate. Your actual adult height may be more or less than this.

Tall Tales and Short Stories

In your mother or grandmother's day, girls often thought being tall was a problem. Today we rarely hear from girls unhappy about being "too tall." Lots of tall women are successful and people look up to them in more ways than one. Tall women can succeed not only in sports like basketball, but also in business and even the movies. For example, Uma Thurman and Geena Davis are both six feet tall. Many tall girls take pride in their height. Here's what one tall girl had to say:

> I've always been the tallest in my class and I like it. My older sister was even taller than me when she was my age. She is the prettiest girl I know. Her boyfriend is shorter than she is, but they don't care.
>
> —MELINDA, AGE 15

We hear more complaints from girls who are shorter than average. Often, their complaints aren't about how *they* feel about being "too short." Rather, they complain about other people's reactions. Let's face it, people think little things are cute. Babies are cute. Fuzzy little dogs that fit on your lap are cute. Too often short people get treated like cute little things. They're not taken seriously. They may be treated like children. They don't always get the respect they deserve. Here's one girl's "short story":

> I'm small and I'm a very fast runner. My cousin used to call me runt and make me cry, but I won all-city honors in track this year. They don't call me runt anymore.
>
> —LIZZIE, AGE 14

The fact is, you can't do much about your height, but you *can* do something about the way you deal with it. You can go out there and be all the other things you want to be. You don't have to be six feet tall to be a good friend. There are no height requirements when it comes to being funny, or smart, or a good athlete. You may not be able to change your height, but you can still achieve your goals!

Feet First

You get taller because the height spurt makes the bones in the trunk of your body and legs grow longer. Some bones start the growth spurt before others, though. The bones in your feet start to grow before other bones. Your feet reach their adult size before you've reached your adult height. Many girls worry about this. They shouldn't. The rest of their bodies will eventually catch up to their feet. As one girl explained:

> I was just a little over five feet tall when I was eleven, but I wore a size eight shoe. I thought, "Oh, no, if my feet keep on growing, they're gonna be gigantic!" I'm sixteen now. I'm five feet eight inches tall, but my feet are still size eight.
>
> —MYRA, AGE 16

Another girl who had Myra's experience said:

I'm sure glad to hear that. I wear a size eight and a half now. I'm only twelve years old and five foot one and a half. People are always teasing me about my big feet. The last time I got tennis shoes, the guy in the store made some joke—If my feet got any bigger, he'd have to sell me the shoe boxes to wear.

I pretended to laugh, but I was embarrassed. I worried maybe my feet were just going to keep getting bigger and bigger.

—LISA, AGE 12

YOUR CHANGING SHAPE

If growing up were simply a matter of getting bigger, adults would look like giant babies. (We may *act* like big babies at times, but adults don't *look* like big babies.) However, some parts of our bodies grow more than others, so that our body *proportions* change. In other words, there's a change in the size of certain parts in relation to other parts.

The drawing of the adult woman and the baby in Figure 25 shows them both at the same height. This makes it easier to see how body proportions change. For example, the baby's head is large compared to other parts of her body. It accounts for one-fourth of her total size, but the woman's head accounts for only one-eighth of her height. Look, too, at how wide the head is compared to the shoulders. On the baby, the head is nearly as wide as the shoulders. On the woman, the head is nowhere near as broad as her shoulders. Also, the woman's legs account for nearly half her height. The baby's legs are a much smaller part of her total size.

---

proportions (pruh-POR-shuns)

GROWING PAINS AND SCOLIOSIS

Growing pains can be a real pain! They're not serious, but they're not much fun either. They are most common in ten- and eleven-year-olds, but younger and older girls also have them.

The pains are not constant. They come and go. They are a dull achy pain. They're often felt behind the knee, in the thigh, or along the shin. They may also occur in the arms, back, groin, shoulders, or ankles. Doctors don't really know what causes growing pains.

Growing pains usually don't need medical treatment. They eventually go away on their own. Until they do, massages, a heating pad, and a nonaspirin pain reliever should help. If the pain is severe or doesn't go away, check it out with a doctor—just to make sure the pain isn't due to something more serious.

Scoliosis is another "growing" problem. It's an abnormal curve in the spine. It's not like the slumped-forward kind of curve from poor posture. Rather, the curve is to the left or right and may result in one hip or shoulder being higher than the other. Or the curve may have an "S" shape. Sometimes, one shoulder blade stands out, or the body has a kind of list. Scoliosis tends to run in families, but, in most cases, the cause is not known.

Many cases are very mild and don't require more than some simple exercises. Even if the exercises can't correct the actual curvature, they can help get rid of the pain that can result from the body being thrown out of balance by the curvature. In serious cases, treatment may require wearing a back brace for a time. Today these braces are light and less bulky than in the past. They can be worn under clothing so they don't show.

Scoliosis is easiest to correct if it is treated early. It's best to start checking for the first signs before puberty begins. In some grade schools, this is done by a school doctor. If it's not done at your school, ask your doctor to check your spine.

---

scoliosis (skoh-lee-OH-sis)

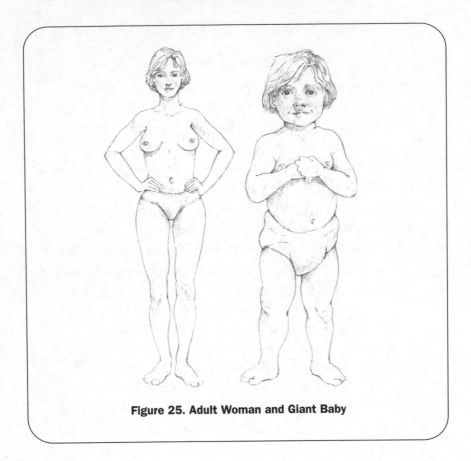

Figure 25. Adult Woman and Giant Baby

The growth spurt also increases the size of your pelvic bones. And the weight spurt deposits fat around the hips. (We'll talk more about that in the next section.) Both these things make your hips wider. As a result, your waist seems narrower in comparison. This, along with breast development, gives you a curvier, more womanly figure.

The growth spurt even changes your face. The lower part of your face gets longer and your chin juts out more. Your hairline moves further back and your forehead widens. As a result, your face is longer, narrower, and less pudgy than when you were a kid.

Because you see yourself in the mirror each day, these changes may not be obvious to you, but look at class pictures over a few years and you'll see the change. Of course, face changes are more dramatic in some girls than in others.

THE WEIGHT SPURT

During your puberty growth spurt, you get heavier as well as taller. In fact, during puberty, girls have what is one of the greatest increases in weight in their lives. This is partly due to the growth of bones, muscles, and internal organs. The extra fat tissue girls gain also adds to their weight.

Like the height spurt, the *weight spurt* lasts about three years. Then the rate at which you gain weight slows back down. During the weight spurt, a girl may gain fifteen pounds or more in a single year. Over the course of the entire weight spurt, the average weight gain is about forty-five pounds. Of course, few of us are exactly average, so you may gain more or less than this, but most girls will add between thirty-five and fifty-five pounds during their weight spurt.

"Too Fat"

Many girls your age are unhappy about their weight. Does that mean most girls are overweight? The answer is no. Only one or two girls out of ten is actually overweight, yet as many as eight out of ten girls think they're "too fat" and would like to lose weight.

Why do so many girls think they're overweight when they're not? For one thing, they forget about the puberty weight spurt. When they suddenly put on a lot of weight they think they're too fat. But you're *supposed* to gain weight during puberty. Also, sometimes girls compare themselves to classmates who are at a different stage of development. If you are near the end of your weight spurt, you can expect to be heavier than a girl who hasn't yet started hers.

The weight spurt and height spurt don't always go hand in hand. They usually happen about the same time, but they don't usually come at *exactly* the same time. It's a kind of seesaw thing. There may be times when you're putting on pounds faster than you're adding inches, and vice versa. As a result, there may be times when you're temporarily chubbier or thinner than usual.

Girls who are having a chubby phase sometimes freak out. They decide they have to start dieting or they'll be fat forever. But, as we'll see later in this chapter, dieting can be hazardous to your health. It can be especially dangerous during puberty!

Basic Body Types

Many girls think they're overweight because they don't understand about body types. There are three basic body types. (See Figure 26.)

- ENDOMORPHS tend to have rounder bodies with more body fat and softer curves.

- ECTOMORPHS are slim, less curvy, and more angular.

- MESOMORPHS are muscular, with wide shoulders and slim hips.

If you're an endomorph, it's important for you to know that your body is meant to be rounder. You may be at your own ideal

---

endomorphs (EN-doe-morfs)
ectomorphs (ECK-toe-morfs)
mesomorphs (MEZ-oh-morfs)

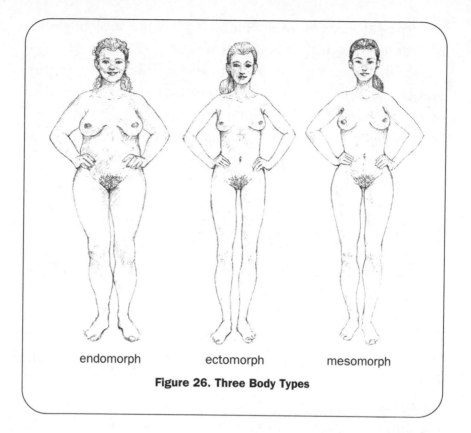

endomorph   ectomorph   mesomorph

Figure 26. Three Body Types

weight, yet look heavier than your friends or classmates who are ectomorphs. Also, the super-skinny models in magazines and on TV may have a more angular body type than yours. If that's the case, you can never really look like they do. It doesn't matter how much weight you lose. So, before you jump to the conclusion that you're "too fat," take your basic body type into account.

The Cult of Thinness

We all see super-skinny models in magazines, and very slender actresses on TV and in movies. All these images of "thinness" can't help influencing us. We may even dream about looking like them. But many of the models and actresses we admire are actually underweight. Even for their slim body type, they may be twenty pounds or so below their healthiest weight.

Still, our society places great value on thinness. This puts pressure on all of us to lose weight. For some young women, this pressure can lead to serious eating disorders (see page 98). Others feel a nagging anxiety about their appearance. You may feel this anxiety even if your weight is perfectly normal and healthy for your body type.

Dieting Can Be Dangerous to Your Health

To lose weight, many girls turn to some kind of fad diet. These diets all promise the same thing: Do something weird with the way you eat and you will lose weight quickly. But fad, or crash, diets almost never work in the long run. You just gain the weight back and often put on more in the process. Something like nine out of ten dieters regain whatever weight they lost. Worst of all, these diets can be downright unhealthy. In fact, any kind of dieting can be dangerous during puberty. At this time in your life, your body is growing rapidly. You need enough nutrients, like vitamins and minerals and proteins, to support this growth.

You need minerals, such as *calcium* and *zinc*, to support the growth of your bones. You also need vitamins such as vitamin D, to carry the calcium to the bones. Remember, this is the time when your bones are supposed to be growing longer, thicker, and stronger. Not getting enough minerals and vitamins can permanently weaken your bones and stunt your growth.

Building strong bones during puberty is important not just for now but for later. The bone mass you develop now must last you for the rest of your life. Beginning at about age twenty-five, women

---

calcium (KAL-see-um)
zinc (ZINK)

start to lose bone mass. The process continues slowly for many, many years. If you don't build up enough bone mass during puberty, your bones may grow weak and fragile as you age. You may eventually develop the disease called *osteoporosis*. Perhaps you've seen old women with stooped posture or "widow's hump." This is a result of osteoporosis. This disease can cause painful fractures of the bones in the spinal column, hips, and elsewhere in the body. Hip fractures are often fatal in the elderly. Building strong bones during puberty helps ensure a longer, healthier, pain-free life when you're older.

Dieting can also slow a girl's development during puberty. Girls who diet to extremes can delay their development by two years or more.

Diets in which you restrict the amount of food you eat too severely or eat only certain kinds of food don't work. Such diets can rob your body of essential nutrients and leave you feeling hungry. Feeling deprived, you're likely to overeat when you stop dieting, so you quickly regain the weight you just lost. Later you start dieting again.

We won't be surprised if this pattern of dieting and overeating and dieting again sounds familiar to you. It happens to a lot of girls and many women, too. It's an unhealthy pattern and can lead to the very serious eating disorders known as *anorexia* and *bulimia*. (See the box on page 98.)

There are ways to lose weight safely, but no girl should diet during puberty unless she first sees her doctor. Your doctor can help you decide how much (if any) weight you need to lose and how to lose it safely. If you are overweight, you and your doctor can work out a balanced diet and exercise program to help you reach a healthier weight.

---

osteoporosis (ah-stee-oh-por-OH-sis)
anorexia (an-oh-REX-ee-uh)
bulimia (boo-LEE-mee-uh)

ANOREXIA AND BULIMIA

Anorexia and *bulimia* are eating disorders. They grow out of an abnormal concern with thinness and weight control. These problems usually start in the teen years. They affect many more girls than boys.

A girl with anorexia eats so little food that she starves herself. She becomes extremely underweight and her body lacks the nutrients needed for normal growth. A person with anorexia will often over-exercise to lose even more weight. Anorexia is a very serious illness. It can lead to severe heart and kidney problems and eventually even death.

Girls with bulimia are often average or slightly above average in weight. They binge (eat a large amount of food in a short time), then they purge (make themselves vomit) to avoid weight gain. People with bulimia often misuse laxatives and diuretics in an attempt to lose weight. Laxatives move food through the body quickly, so fewer calories are absorbed. Diuretics, or "water pills," draw water from the body and make you urinate more. A girl with bulimia may develop digestive and dental problems, ulcers, and serious heart disorders.

People with eating disorders need professional help. Most experts believe that psychological factors play a major role in causing these disorders. Treatment usually requires counseling or group therapy, and often a hospital stay.

If you need help with an eating disorder, talk to an adult you trust. You'll also find useful resources at the back of this book.

If you have a friend with a secret eating disorder, the best thing you can do is to tell an adult. Maybe you promised not to tell, but this is one of those times when you should break your promise and get help for your friend. Otherwise you may be allowing your friend to put herself in real danger.

---

diuretics (die-yur-ET-icks)

TAKING CARE OF YOUR BODY

Eating Right and Exercising

To grow, your body needs enough of many different nutrients. To get all the nutrients you need, you must eat a variety of foods from each food group: grains, vegetables, fruits, milk and meat, and beans. What food and how much food should you eat from each group? There's not one answer for everybody. It depends on your age and your level of activity. Find out what's right for you. Visit www.mypyramid.gov/kids. Find the list of subjects on the left side of the screen. Then go to "My Pyramid Plan." On the next screen enter your age, sex, and physical activity. Then hit "submit." The next screen tells you how much of each type of food you should eat.

We have already talked about the importance of calcium for healthy bones. Studies show that girls are likely to get only half, or less, of the calcium they need in their diet. Be especially careful to eat foods that are rich in calcium. These include calcium-fortified nonfat milk, calcium-fortified soy milk, yogurt, cheese, other dairy products, calcium-fortified cereals, calcium-fortified orange juice, broccoli, kale, green beans, and tofu. Teenagers should get at least 1300 milligrams of calcium daily. An eight-ounce glass of fortified nonfat milk contains about 300 milligrams. Fortified orange juice usually provides about the same amount of calcium as fortified nonfat milk. (It's easy to know which foods are calcium-fortified because the packages say so—usually in large type.) If you can't drink milk or don't like it, ask your doctor about a supplement to make sure you get that all-important calcium.

Besides eating right, we all need regular exercise. Because your heart and lungs grow larger during puberty, your body can handle more exercise. And it *needs* it. Exercise helps you achieve your best weight. In fact, not exercising may be the most important factor that causes people to be overweight. It may be even more important than overeating, although the two tend to go together.

But exercise is more than just a tool to help you keep your tummy flat and your weight down. Exercise strengthens your heart, increases your energy level, and sends more *oxygen* to all parts of your body. Exercise also helps deposit calcium in the bones. This is especially important during your teens. This is when you are building up the bone mass that will sustain you for the rest of your life.

After reading about all these benefits from exercise, you may be thinking that you should go out and jog for twelve hours a day, but too much exercise can be bad. The combination of too much exercise and improper diet can be especially harmful. (See the box on "Female Athletic Syndrome.")

Tobacco, Alcohol, and Other Drugs

You can't grow a healthy body if you're using drugs, alcohol, or tobacco. You've probably already learned in school about the dangers of these substances. It's especially important to avoid using them during puberty when your body is growing. Alcohol, for example, robs the body of zinc, which you need for growing strong bones.

You may feel a lot of peer pressure to use tobacco, drugs, or alcohol. In addition to peer pressure, you must also resist advertisers' efforts to get you to use alcohol or tobacco. You probably know that tobacco is habit-forming. It can be very hard to stop smoking once you've started. You may even know that most smokers start during their teens. No wonder the giant tobacco companies have aimed so much advertising at young people. From their point of view, your teen years are important. They are

---

oxygen (OX-suh-jin)

FEMALE ATHLETIC SYNDROME

The *Female Athletic Syndrome* is also called FAS, for short, or *Female Athletic Triad*. It is a group of problems that can affect girls who are athletes. It most often affects girls who participate in activities such as gymnastics, long-distance running, or ballet dancing. To win at these sports or become a ballerina, girls must have very lean bodies and train hard. To keep their weight down, many of these girls go on crash diets, use diet pills, laxatives, or diuretics, or vomit after eating. Some develop the eating disorders discussed in the box on page 98.

Low weight, combined with the long hours of exercise, can delay puberty. Girls who have already started puberty and have had their first periods may stop menstruating altogether. The menstrual periods usually start again once the girl gains some weight and cuts back her training. However, the effect on her bones may be permanent. The combination of eating problems and delayed puberty or stopping of menstruation causes bone problems. As a result a girl may never attain her normal adult height. Other bones may be so weakened that they break easily. Some girls even develop osteoporosis, the "brittle bone" disease usually seen only in elderly women.

If you are an athlete, you need to be aware of FAS. If you are eating improperly in order to get your weight down, you may be at risk for eating disorders. Talk with your coach and doctor about the problem. If you have started menstruating and then miss three periods in a row, you should see a doctor who specializes in taking care of athletes. Ask your coach to recommend one. If you have not begun to develop breasts or pubic hair or had your first period by the expected ages, you, too, should see your doctor.

The American College of Sports Medicine advises the following steps for treating FAS: a 5 to 15 percent reduction in training, a 5 to 20 percent increase in calories, and a weight gain of 2 to 10 pounds. For more information on FAS, see the Resource Section at the back of this book.

the years when they have the best chance to hook you as a long-term smoker. Studies show that people who have a healthy lifestyle during their teen years tend to stay fit for their entire lives. Not using alcohol, tobacco, or drugs, and eating right and getting regular exercise are the keys to that healthy lifestyle.

LIKING THE WAY YOU LOOK

A healthy body is a good body in our book. It would be nice if we could all just look at our bodies and say, "Hey, I like the way I look," but we live in a society where competition is a way of life. People compete, companies compete, even countries compete. We are always comparing and competing to see who's best. But who decides what's best?

Most of us get our ideas about what's the "best" or "most attractive" kind of female body from supermodels and actresses. We see these "perfect" women everywhere—in magazines, on billboards, in movies, and on TV. Their teeth, hair, and eyes sparkle and shine. They are usually tall and always very thin. Often they are blond, blue-eyed, and white-skinned. They have flat stomachs, tiny waists, and long legs. Their skin is smooth and glowing. They have no pimples or freckles, no hair on their legs or underarms, and not a single bulge or blemish.

As you may have noticed, there are few of us who actually look like this. For one thing, we aren't all thin with tiny waists, flat tummies, and firm thighs. Our hair gets mussed and tangled and may not have much shine even on a good hair day. Our clothes get rumpled and wrinkled and our faces may, too. And we aren't all white-skinned, blond-haired, and blue-eyed.

Yet, everywhere we turn, we see images of "perfect" women. We drive across town, ride a bus, or go to a show, and there they are. Larger than life, they peer down at us from billboards and movie screens. Turn the pages of a magazine. There they are, airbrushed into perfection. Flip the TV channel. There they are again, with their "perfect" bodies, leading glamorous, apparently problem-free lives.

By the time a girl reaches puberty, how many images of perfection have passed before her eyes? Counting all the books, magazines, movies, and TV shows she's ever seen, what's it come to—a million, ten million? Who knows, maybe more.

It's no wonder that so many of us start to feel there is something about our shape, or face, or skin, or hair that is somehow not

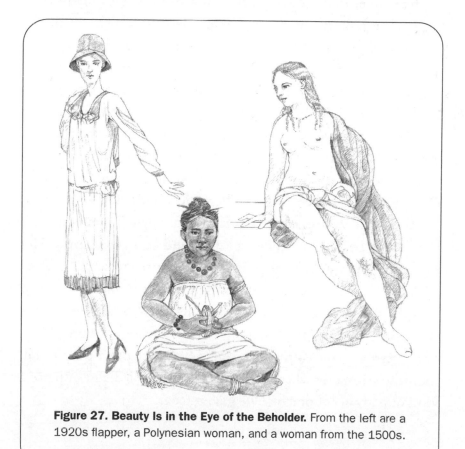

Figure 27. Beauty Is in the Eye of the Beholder. From the left are a 1920s flapper, a Polynesian woman, and a woman from the 1500s.

right. Our real-life bodies don't look like all these perfect bodies, so we feel unhappy about ourselves. This is, of course, just the way the people who spend so much money creating these images want us to feel. They want women to spend millions and millions of dollars each year to "improve" their looks. And we do. We buy hair dyes, makeup, diet products, leg and underarm hair removers, tummy flatteners, breast developers, waist trimmers, and on and on. Some people even have operations to make their tummies flatter, their noses straighter, or their breasts a different size.

Do you sometimes feel unhappy about the way you look? If so, remember that these perfect bodies seem better only because they are in fashion. What's in fashion depends on the particular culture and the particular time. The drawings you see in Figure 27 show bodies that have been in fashion at other times and in other cultures. The first drawing is a flapper from America in the 1920s. Back then, curvy bodies and big breasts were definitely not in fashion. In fact, women with big breasts wrapped them tightly so they wouldn't stick out. The drawing on the right shows a woman from Europe in the 1500s. Today she would be considered a bit chunky, but back then hers was the perfect body. The third drawing shows a Polynesian woman. She hardly matches our culture's standard of beauty, but in her culture, she'd be a great beauty. Her rounded body would be the best and most attractive.

Learning to appreciate yourself and to love your own body, regardless of whether it matches up with what's in fashion, is a big step in growing up. It's also a big step in becoming more attractive, because if you learn to like your own looks, other people will, too. It won't matter whether you have the so-called best or perfect kind of body—not one bit. We guarantee it.

5.

BODY HAIR, PERSPIRATION, PIMPLES, AND OTHER CHANGES

During puberty, hair starts to grow in places where it never grew before. You grow pubic hair and underarm hair. Darker hair may grow on your arms and legs as well. Puberty also affects our sweat and oil glands. We perspire more and develop an adult body odor. Oil glands in our scalp are more active. They make more oil and that makes your hair oilier. Oil glands in the skin also work over-time. Sometimes the extra oil they make gets trapped and the result is a faceful of pimples.

Let's face it, some of the changes we talk about in this chapter are not a lot of fun. Over the years, we've seen many girls excited about starting puberty. They can't wait to develop breasts and have their first period. But we've yet to come across a girl who "couldn't wait" to get her first pimple.

Zits and body odor are less-than-wonderful parts of puberty. We won't try to pretend otherwise. We won't try to cover it up by talking about how great it is that you're "becoming a woman." Instead, we'll give you some facts, so you know what to expect. We won't leave it at that, though. We'll also tell you about *acne* treatments and how to cope with body odor and unwanted hair.

UNDERARM AND BODY HAIR

Underarm hair may start growing anytime during the puberty years. Some girls are well into puberty before they get it. Other girls start to grow underarm hair about the same time that they start getting pubic hairs or developing breasts. For a few girls, underarm hair is the first outward sign of puberty. On average, girls start growing underarm hair a year or so after pubic hair.

More hair may grow on your arms and legs as you go through puberty. Usually it will be darker than it was when you were younger, but some girls told us the color got lighter again as they got older.

A Hairy Question

In other countries, people think underarm or leg hair on a woman is sexy. In our country, the opposite seems to be true, at least in many people's minds. The pretty, glamorous women in magazines, on TV, and in movies have smooth, hairless legs and armpits. It's not that these women are somehow different from us and don't grow hair in these places. They are hairless because they shave their hair or remove it in some other way.

---

acne (ACK-nee)

Boys usually feel proud when they start growing body hair. It is a sign that they are turning from boys into men. On men, body hair is attractive and manly. On women, it's considered unattractive and not at all feminine. Go figure!

You'll have to decide for yourself about removing hair from your legs and underarms. It's not always easy to decide. Your friends may pressure you, as in this girl's case:

> I wasn't going to shave my legs. Then my girlfriends started saying, "Oh, gross, look at all the hair on your legs. How come you don't shave it?" So I started doing it even though I didn't really want to.
>
> —PATRICIA, AGE 15

Other girls want to shave their legs, but their mothers say no. If that's your problem, you and your mom will have to work it out. Try explaining *why* you want to shave your legs. Better yet, write your reasons in a letter to your mom. This is often the best way to make your case.

Besides removing hair from their underarms and legs, females also remove unwanted hair from their upper lips, other parts of the face, or from the "bikini line." In the following pages, you'll learn about the different ways of removing unwanted hair.

SHAVING AND OTHER WAYS OF DEALING WITH UNWANTED HAIR

Shaving is the most popular method of removing unwanted hair. It's cheap, easy, and fairly safe, though you may nick yourself a lot before you learn how to do it. Shaving works well for leg, underarm, and bikini-line hair. There's one big drawback, though. Hair regrows quickly. To stay smooth, women usually need to shave every two or three days.

The chart on pages 110–111 lists other methods of dealing with unwanted hair. However, you shouldn't shave or use any of these other methods if

- you have cuts, rashes, bumps, or breaks in the skin.

- your skin is sunburned.

- you plan to swim or use sunscreen in the next twenty-four hours.

Razors: A Buyer's Guide

You have a choice of blade or electric razors. Some women prefer electrics, especially the wet/dry razors you can use in the shower. You're less likely to cut yourself with an electric razor, but a good electric razor isn't cheap. And it won't give you as close a shave as a blade razor will.

DOES IT REALLY GROW BACK THICKER AND DARKER?

No, shaving doesn't really make hair grow back thicker and darker. It may look that way, though.

Hairs taper to a point at the end. The hair shaft is thinner at the tip than in the middle or at the root. Shaving cuts the hair in its thickest part. (See Figure 28.)

If you've never shaved, much of what's visible above the skin's surface is the thin, tapered part of each shaft. Once you shave, the thin, tapered tips are gone. All you see is the thickest part of each hair shaft. Your hair isn't really any thicker. Sure looks that way, though.

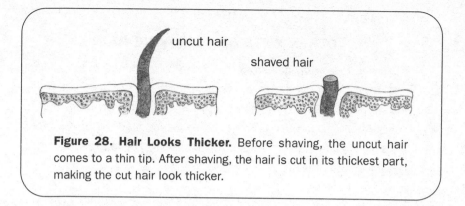

Figure 28. Hair Looks Thicker. Before shaving, the uncut hair comes to a thin tip. After shaving, the hair is cut in its thickest part, making the cut hair look thicker.

Most women choose blade razors. The two most popular types are the disposable and the cartridge razors. With one, you throw the entire razor away when the blade gets dull. With the other, you discard the blade cartridge, but keep the rest of the razor for use with a new cartridge.

You also have a choice of single- or twin- or even triple-blade razors. You'll probably like the closer shave you get from a twin- or triple-blade razor, but you are less likely to cut yourself with a single-blade. Twin- or triple-blade razors are more likely to cause ingrown hairs. If you're prone to ingrown hairs, go for the single-blade razor.

There are also razors made specially for women and razors with pivoting heads or other special features, but these special features didn't make much difference to women in tests done by Consumer Reports. Razors with a lubricating strip did, however, get better ratings.

Shaving Tips for Blade Razors

These tips should help you shave smoothly and safely.

- MAKE SURE YOUR BLADES ARE CLEAN, SHARP, AND FREE OF NICKS. Change blades at least every four or five shaves. A

OTHER WAYS OF REMOVING HAIR

Read and follow any directions that come with these products. Don't use more often or longer than recommended. If there are chemicals in the product, always do a skin patch test. Wait twenty-four hours to check results. Don't use products on your face, underarms, or genital area unless the directions specifically say so. These areas are more sensitive than others.

BLEACHING: Removes color from hair, so it's less visible; lasts up to four weeks; used on upper lip, arms, and legs.

Drawbacks: Not good for thick growth; doesn't actually remove hair.

To avoid problems: Never use household bleach or any product that isn't made specifically for hair in the area you want to bleach.

TWEEZING: Plucks out hair to the root; lasts for weeks; used on eyebrows and stray facial or breast hairs.

Drawbacks: Often too painful for lips or breasts; not useful for large areas or thick growth.

To avoid problems: First soften skin with a light moisturizer; tweeze in direction of hair growth; swab with a nonalcohol skin tonic after every few yanks.

EPILATING: Looks like an electric razor; works like a set of tiny tweezers; lasts for several weeks; good for large areas like legs.

Drawbacks: Often painful; unit costs up to $150; risk of ingrown hair, especially on the face; don't use on face.

To avoid problems: Use a buff puff or similar product before and after using the epilating machine.

DEPILATION: Using creams, lotions, or gels to dissolve hair; depilatories are applied in the direction of hair growth and wiped or rinsed away after a specified time; lasts longer than shaving; used on upper lip, legs, or bikini line.

---

epilating (EP-uh-late-ing)
depilation (depp-uh-LAY-shun)
depilatories (de-PILL-uh-tor-eez)

Drawbacks: Can cause skin irritation and infection; too irritating for many women.

To avoid problems: Don't use for a week after using Retin-A, buff puff, or any other products that remove loose dead cells from the surface of skin.

WAXING: Done in salons or at home; cold wax strips are pressed—or heated wax is spread—on the skin in the direction of hair growth; wax is torn off (like a Band-Aid), ripping out the hairs caught in the wax; lasts several weeks; used on legs, bikini line, upper lip, underarms, and eyebrows; safest if done at a salon.

Drawbacks: Painful; hair must be at least one-quarter inch long, so there's stubble between treatments; can cause irritation, infection, or ingrown hairs; may discolor skin for months; uneven heating of wax in microwaves can cause skin burns.

To avoid problems: Apply cold compress to treated area; don't use over warts, moles, and varicose veins; don't use if you are prone to infection or have diabetes or circulatory problems.

ELECTROLYSIS: Uses electric current to destroy hair roots; a permanent method, though some hair may grow back; usually requires a trained operator, though now there are tweezer electrolysis kits for home use; self-treatment is not recommended for areas that can be seen only with a mirror.

Drawbacks: Expensive and time-consuming; may be painful; may result in infection or scarring if done improperly.

To avoid problems: Check that the operator uses sterilized needles and disposable gloves; skin should be cleaned with an antiseptic first; call your doctor or the International Guild of Professional Electrologists (800-830-3247) for a referral to a trained, licensed professional (thirty-one states require licenses); before self-treating, ask a professional to show you how.

---

electrolysis (e-lek-TROL-uh-sis)

REMOVING HAIR AT THE BIKINI LINE

Girls who wear bikinis or high-cut bathing suits don't want pubic hair to show, but removing pubic hair can cause problems if it isn't done carefully. Here's some info about removing hair at the bikini line.

Plucking pubic hair can cause bumps and skin irritation. It might be okay for a few stray hairs, but removing more than a few this way is too painful and takes too much time.

Some creams can be used in the bikini area, as long as you follow directions carefully. Make sure the product is made for use on this area of the body. Always do a skin patch test first. Wait twenty-four hours to check the results.

You can shave your bikini line with a razor, but go easy. Use plenty of shaving cream. Always shave down, in the direction of hair growth. Try not to go over and over the same area. Even when you're careful, you may find that shaving leaves unsightly red bumps and irritated skin. This problem is especially common among African-American women. (See box on page 122.) Test first by shaving a small area. Then wait at least twenty-four hours to check your skin.

There are also wax kits for use on the bikini line. Make sure you use a wax that is labeled safe for use on the bikini line. Even so, you may have small red dots for a day or so after waxing.

dull blade will pull, or drag, on your skin. This causes a painful rash called razor burn. Dropping a razor can cause hard-to-see nicks in the blade. If you drop it, chuck it!

• WET THE HAIR FIRST. Give the hair at least three minutes to soak up the water. Warm water expands and softens hair, making it easier to cut and reducing razor drag. Don't soak for more than fifteen minutes, though. After that, the skin plumps up. Then you're more likely to cut yourself and less likely to get a close shave.

- USE SHAVING CREAM OR GEL, NOT SOAP. Creams and gels reduce the drag of the razor on your skin. They also soften the hair. Soap dulls blades and hardens hair, making shaving more difficult.

- GO EASY AND RINSE OFTEN. Don't mash the razor into your skin. Use a light touch. Try not to go over and over the same area. Rinse your razor often to keep the blade free of hair.

- SHAVE IN THE RIGHT DIRECTION. Shaving against the direction of hair growth gives the closest shave. Shaving in the direction of hair growth is easier on the skin, though. On the legs, you can shave upward, against the hair growth. But on the underarms and other sensitive areas, shave in the direction of hair growth.

- RINSE WITH COOL WATER AND PAT DRY. Rinsing with cool water closes pores and soothes skin. Pat, rather than rub, dry. You can use soothing lotions. Look for ones with aloe vera. Don't use lotions with perfume or alcohol. Don't use underarm deodorants right after shaving.

- NEVER LEND OR BORROW A RAZOR. Don't share. You risk sharing an infection.

PERSPIRATION AND BODY ODOR

You run up and down the stairs ten times in a row. Or maybe it's just a sizzling hot summer day. What happens? You sweat, of course. When temperatures soar or you work out, your sweat glands swing into action. They pour out the sweat. (Stress, fear, and other strong emotions can also trigger your sweat glands.)

You have millions of sweat glands. They're in nearly every inch of skin on your body. They keep you from overheating by pouring out sweat. Sweat is 99 percent water, with a little bit of salt thrown into the mix. The water quickly evaporates, cooling you down. And the salt in the sweat helps draw more water from your body.

During puberty, the output from your sweat glands increases, and special sweat glands in your underarms and genital area become active for the first time. This means you sweat more and in more places. You may notice more sweat on your forehead, upper lip, neck, and chest when you exercise. Fear or worry, on the other hand, usually causes sweat in the armpits, palms, and soles of your feet. Even if you're fearless and worry-free, you'll probably sweat a lot in these areas. The reason: These areas have more sweat glands than other parts of the body.

Your body odor also changes during puberty. Sweat, by itself, doesn't cause an unpleasant odor. It is nearly odorless. But bacteria that live on human skin break the sweat down, and this causes an odor. These bacteria particularly like sweat from those special glands in your armpits and genital area that get activated during puberty.

Most of what we call body odor comes from the armpits. Here there are the special glands that bacteria like, as well as warm, moist conditions that are perfect for breeding bacteria. And sweat can get really stinky when bacteria have time to go to work.

Dealing with Perspiration and Body Odor

Puberty changes in body odor and *perspiration* (sweat) are natural and healthy. It's all a part of growing up. Still, some young people worry about odor and sweating. This isn't really too surprising.

---

perspiration (pur-spuh-RAY-shun)

Companies spend millions of dollars on TV commercials and magazine ads to make us worry about body odor and staying dry.

Don't let them make you uptight about your body! Sweating is good for you. It keeps you from frying! It's also your body's way of getting rid of waste products. However, there's no reason you have to be smelly even if you sweat a lot. It's easy to keep yourself smelling clean and fresh. Here are a few tips.

- BATHE OR SHOWER REGULARLY. Daily washing rinses away the bacteria that cause odor. It's especially important to wash your underarms and vulva.

- USE AN ANTIBACTERIAL SOAP UNDER YOUR ARMS. Studies show that these soaps can control bacteria for up to sixteen hours.

- WEAR FRESHLY LAUNDERED CLOTHING. The bacteria that cause odor can hang around in your clothes. Keep them clean.

- WEAR CLOTHES THAT "BREATHE." If you perspire quite a bit, try wearing 100 percent cotton underwear. Cotton absorbs more and allows air to circulate, keeping you dry.

Deodorants and Antiperspirants

If the odor or amount of your underarm perspiration bothers you, you may want to use a *deodorant* or an *antiperspirant*. Many deodorants cover up body odor with a scent of their own. Some also fight the bacteria that cause the odor. Antiperspirants keep you dry by cutting down on the amount of perspiration. Most deodorants also contain an antiperspirant.

---

antibacterial (ann-tee-back-TEER-ee-uhl)
deodorant (dee-OH-duh-runt)
antiperspirant (ann-tee-PUR-spuh-runt)

FEMININE HYGIENE SPRAY

Feminine hygiene sprays are made for use on the vulva. We don't recommend them. They can cause irritation. Besides, unless you have an infection, your vulva area shouldn't have an unpleasant smell. It isn't hard to smell fresh. Washing daily with soap and water and putting on clean cotton underwear each day should be all it takes.

If your vulva smells bad, you may have an infection. You should see a doctor rather than cover up these odors with a deodorant spray.

These products come in sprays, sticks, gels, creams, lotions, and roll-ons. Some are unscented, and some have a scent added. Some are advertised as being especially for women, but there really isn't much difference between a "man's deodorant" and a "woman's deodorant."

Antiperspirants contain some form of *aluminum*. Some experts feel even the small amount of aluminum that could enter the body in this way is unsafe. Other experts say just the opposite. The government sides with those who say it's safe. If you're worried, use a deodorant without aluminum. Or, if you feel you need an antiperspirant, use one with *buffered* aluminum *sulfate*, which isn't easily absorbed beyond the skin's outer layers.

Whatever product you decide to use, do read the directions. Some products should be applied right after you bathe, while you're still damp. Dampness activates the wetness- and bacteria-fighting ingredients. Other products work best when you use

---

aluminum (uh-LOO-muh-num)
buffered (BUFF-erd)
sulfate (SUL-fate)

them at bedtime rather than first thing in the morning. If you perspire a lot, try using an antiperspirant both before bedtime and before you get dressed in the morning.

PIMPLES, ACNE, AND OTHER SKIN PROBLEMS

Zits are a fact of life for most girls during puberty. Oil glands in the skin become active—too active. The extra oil they make often gets trapped behind blocked pores. The result can be a faceful of pimples.

What Causes Acne?

Acne is the term doctors use for what we call zits, pimples, whiteheads, and blackheads. Doctors call all these skin problems acne because they all start with oil glands and clogged pores.

We have oil glands all over our bodies. They are most common on the face, neck, chest, and back. This is also where acne is most likely to strike.

Figure 29 shows a hair follicle and oil gland. Hair follicles lie below the skin's surface. Every hair on your body has its own follicle. In the lower part of each follicle there's an oil gland. These glands make an oil called *sebum*. The sebum flows from the gland and along the hair shaft. It comes out the opening, or pore, in the skin's surface. As the sebum flows out, it carries away dead skin cells from the walls of the hair follicle.

Puberty affects your hair follicles and oil glands in several ways. The glands make more sebum than ever before. More skin cells come off the wall of the hair follicles. The dead skin cells also tend to stick together more than they did before puberty. These sticky cells can clump together and form a plug that blocks the pore.

---

sebum (SEE-bum)

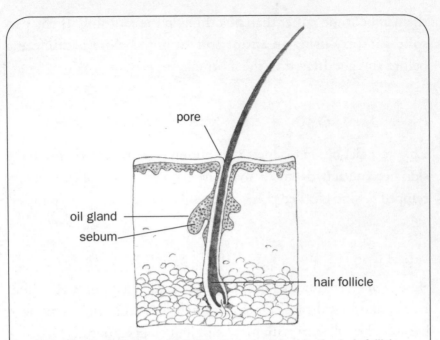

Figure 29. Follicle and Oil Gland. A gland inside the hair follicle makes an oil called sebum. Normally the pore of the hair follicle is unblocked, allowing the sebum to slowly flow out and lubricate the skin.

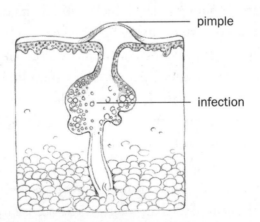

Figure 30. A Pimple. If the pore and upper part of the hair follicle become blocked, the sebum can't flow out through the pore. The result may be an infection that results in the swelling and redness we call a pimple.

Even though the pore is blocked, the oil gland goes right on making sebum. But the sebum can no longer leave the follicle. It collects behind the plug and swells the hair follicle. This shows up as a white bump just below the skin's surface. We call this white bump a whitehead.

Sometimes pressure from the trapped sebum pushes the plug up above the skin's surface. If this happens, you develop a blackhead. The black color is not from dirt trapped in the plug. A chemical reaction on the skin's surface turns the plug black.

Whiteheads and blackheads are milder kinds of acne. Pimples are more serious. They occur when bacteria infect the trapped sebum. Bacteria that are harmless when they live on the skin's surface cause the infection. When they get into the sebum trapped behind a blocked pore these "harmless" bacteria begin to multiply. This results in the redness and swelling which we call a pimple. (See Figure 30.)

Sometimes the walls inside an infected hair follicle will burst open. The infection then spreads under the skin. This is the most serious kind of acne. It causes large, painful red bumps.

Treatment

Whiteheads, blackheads, pimples, and severe acne are no fun. They're certainly not very attractive. Worse yet, severe acne can cause permanent pitting or scarring of the skin. The good news is the problem can be treated. In fact, there are a number of things you can do on your own. What works best will depend on the type of acne you have and how severe it is.

Some people think acne is caused by poor hygiene. They think washing more often will cure the problem. This isn't true. Washing your face twice a day is usually enough. Washing more often than that can't prevent or cure acne.

Sometimes oil from the hair can irritate acne breakouts on your forehead. In these cases, washing the hair often and wearing it back, away from the forehead, may help. If you have acne, don't use oil-based cosmetics. Look for the words *noncomedogenic* or *nonacnegenic* on the cosmetics you use.

Adults may tell you not to pop your pimples. They're right. It can drive the infection deeper into your skin and leave scars.

Over-the-Counter Treatments

Over-the-counter means you don't need a doctor's prescription. There are many products you can buy for treating acne. If you use one of these products, there are some things you should know.

- BENZOYL PEROXIDE. *Benzoyl peroxide* is the main ingredient in many over-the-counter acne treatments. It attacks the bacteria that cause pimples and acne. It also helps break up the blockage in the pore of the hair follicle. If you use one of these products, go slow at first. Before using the product, test it on a small area of skin to make sure you're not allergic.

  When first using the product, apply it to the infected area only every other day. After a couple of weeks, you can apply it daily. Be careful not to get benzoyl peroxide on your clothes. It's a powerful bleach, which can permanently spot your clothes.

- SALICYLIC ACID. *Salicylic acid* is also effective for treating acne. It comes in various over-the-counter products. It removes whiteheads and blackheads and helps prevent their

---

noncomedogenic (non-cah-mee-doe-JEN-ick)
nonacnegenic (non-ack-nuh-JEN-ick)
benzoyl peroxide (BEN-zoh-il pur-OCK-side)
salicylic (sal-uh-SIL-ick)

ACNE AND FOOD

People used to believe that eating certain foods could cause acne. Chocolate and greasy foods like french fries were the most popular villains. Doctors haven't been able to prove a link between diet and acne. Still, if you find that certain foods give you pimples, it's best to avoid them. You can be sure that eating less fried foods and chocolate won't hurt you!

return. Salicylic acid products can be used with other treatments. Follow the directions that come with the product.

- ABRASIVE SOAPS AND SCRUBS. These can actually make acne worse. Don't use them if you have lots of pimples or severe acne. African-American teenagers should always avoid abrasive soaps or other abrasive products. (See the box on page 122.)

Remember: Any over-the-counter medications for acne may irritate the skin. Always carefully follow the directions. Expect to wait six to eight weeks before seeing results.

Medical Treatment

Some people say, "Just let acne run its course; you just have to grow out of it." But medical treatment can help. Also, serious cases of acne can cause permanent scars if left untreated. If you have anything more than mild acne, you may need to see a doctor. The guidelines below will help you decide. See a doctor if you have acne and any of the following are true.

- You have used an over-the-counter product for two months or more, with little improvement in your skin.

SPECIAL SKIN CONCERNS
FOR AFRICAN-AMERICAN WOMEN

African-American women and other women of color need to be especially careful about the use of hair removal and skin products.

- **Abrasive soaps and scrubs.** Abrasive soaps or scrubs can cause permanent patches of lighter or darker skin. Don't use these products.

- **Razor bumps.** African-American women who shave may be more likely to develop razor bumps. Shaving along the bikini line is especially likely to cause problems. Shaving cuts hair at an angle, leaving a sharp tip. After shaving, curly hair can pull back under the skin's surface or loop over and grow back into the skin. (See Figure 31.) This can cause angry, inflamed bumps on the surface of the skin. If you have this problem, don't shave pubic hair. When shaving elsewhere, always shave in the direction the hair grows.

- **Chemical hair removers.** Be especially careful when you use one of these products. They can irritate. Always test on a small patch of skin before applying to larger areas. Stay out of the sun and don't go swimming for twenty-four hours after use.

- **Keloids.** African-American skin is more likely to form abnormal scars known as keloids. If you're subject to keloids, even a little nick from shaving or popping a pimple could leave a noticeable scar. Talk to your doctor before using any method of hair removal.

---

keloid (KEY-loyd)

- Your acne keeps you from fully enjoying your life.

- You have large, red, and painful acne bumps.

- You are dark-skinned and have noticed that acne is causing dark patches on your skin.

- Severe cases of acne run in your family.

- You are only nine or ten years old when acne first appears.

Your doctor can prescribe a treatment that fits your acne problem. He or she can also prescribe drugs that you can't buy over-the-counter. Always be careful to follow all the directions your doctor gives you. Be sure to tell your doctor about any over-the-counter products you may have used or are now using. Some products may cause bad interactions with the doctor's prescription. It may take a couple of months, or more, of treatment to

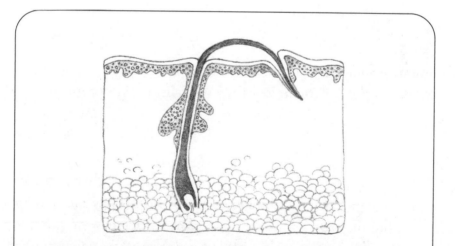

Figure 31. Razor Bumps. This problem happens with tight curly hair. Shaving cuts hair at an angle, leaving a sharp tip. The tip can curl back into the skin, causing a painful bump.

THE UPSIDE OF PUBERTY

Puberty isn't all perspiration and pimples. It can seem that way when we've spent a whole class period (or a whole chapter) on the downside. So, at the end of these classes, we remind everybody there's an upside to puberty by listing all the good things that can happen as you go through puberty. Here's one of those lists. What would you add to it?

more privileges

getting to stay out later

being more my own boss

driving a car

getting into R-rated movies

having my body get curvier

more respect

more allowance

joining the team in
high school

getting my braces off

getting a job

dating

new school

new friends

going to parties

having my own money

going to college

making my own decisions
(sometimes)

improve your acne. In some cases your doctor may refer you to a *dermatologist*. A dermatologist is a specialist in skin problems.

STRETCH MARKS

Some young people develop stretch marks during puberty. Stretch marks are purplish or white lines on the skin. They aren't common, but they can happen if rapid growth stretches the skin too quickly. Sometimes gaining a lot of weight causes stretch marks. Often these marks get much less noticeable as a person gets older.

---

dermatologist (der-muh-TAH-luh-jist)

But other than waiting for them to go away, there's not much you do about them.

Stretch marks, pubic hair, underarm hair, perspiration, and acne are just some of the changes that happen during puberty. In the next chapter, we'll be talking about still others.

6.

THE REPRODUCTIVE ORGANS AND THE MENSTRUAL CYCLE

In Chapter 3, we talked about the sex organs on the outside of the body. We also have sex organs inside our bodies. They're called *reproductive organs*. Why? Because these organs make it possible for us to reproduce—to have babies. In this chapter, we'll talk about these organs and how they change as we go through puberty.

One result of these changes in the reproductive organs is that a girl has her first menstrual period. Another result is that a girl ovulates for the first time. (As you may recall from Chapter 1, the *ovum* is the female reproductive cell. Ova are stored in the ovaries. *Ovulation* is the release of an ovum from the ovary.)

A mature woman ovulates about once a month. About two weeks after she ovulates, she usually has her menstrual period. She repeats this cycle of ovulation and menstruation about every month for much of her adult life. (One exception occurs during pregnancy. A pregnant woman doesn't ovulate.)

This cycle of ovulation and menstruation is called the *menstrual cycle*. Young girls often menstruate without ovulating. It takes a while before they get into a regular cycle of ovulation and menstruation.

In this chapter, you'll learn how your ovaries produce a ripe ovum. We'll explain what happens inside your body when you have your period. You'll learn about the menstrual cycle. We'll also give some guidelines to help you know what's normal, or not normal, throughout your menstrual cycle. Finally, you'll learn about premenstrual syndrome, or *PMS*, and some other menstrual changes you may experience.

THE INSIDE STORY: YOUR REPRODUCTIVE ORGANS

The sex organs inside the female body allow us to reproduce. These organs are listed below. Read the list. Then see if you can find these organs in Figure 32.

THE REPRODUCTIVE ORGANS

- OVARIES: Where the female reproductive cells, the ova (plural of "ovum") are stored.

- UTERINE TUBES: The tubes the ova travel through on their way to the uterus (also called egg tubes, or Fallopian tubes, or just tubes).

- UTERUS: Where a baby grows during the nine months of pregnancy (also called the womb).

Fallopian (fuh-LOH-pee-un)

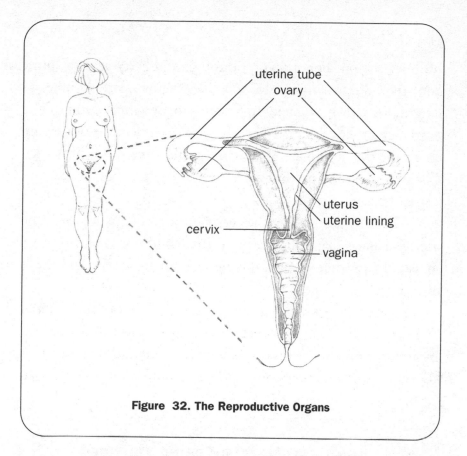

Figure 32. The Reproductive Organs

- **UTERINE LINING:** The thick, bloody lining of the uterus that is shed during each period.

- **CERVIX:** The lower part of the uterus, which protrudes into the top of the vagina.

- **CERVICAL CANAL:** A narrow tunnel in the center of the *cervix;* the *cervical canal* leads from the vagina into the uterus.

- **VAGINA:** A muscular tube inside the body, running from the vulva to the cervix.

---

cervix (SIR-vicks)
cervical (SIR-vick-uhl)

The Inner Growth Spurt

It's not just your bones that go through a puberty growth spurt. Your reproductive organs do, too. The vagina nearly doubles in length. In grown women, it is three to five inches long. The ovaries and tubes also get bigger. In grown women, the ovaries are about the size and shape of a large almond (one still in its shell). The tubes are three to four inches long. They are about as thick as a strand of spaghetti.

The uterus, including the cervix, grows, too. As it grows, the uterus changes shape and position. In a child, the uterus is tube-shaped. In an adult woman, the uterus is about the size and shape of an upside-down pear.

Figure 33 shows the reproductive organs in a young girl and in a woman. As you can see, the uterus is upright before puberty. In grown women, the uterus usually tilts forward, but this isn't always the case. In some women, the uterus doesn't tip forward. In

---

DON'T BELIEVE EVERYTHING YOU SEE

Drawings often make it look as if the vagina is hollow, with empty space inside. Not so! Earlier we explained that the vagina is like a balloon which hasn't been blown up. There's no hollow space inside the vagina. You can also think of the vagina as being like the sleeve of a coat. If the coat isn't being worn and there's nothing inside the sleeve, there won't be a hollow space. Rather, the sides of the empty sleeve will lie flat against each other. There's no empty space inside the vagina either. Normally, the inner walls of the vagina, like the insides of the sleeve, touch each other.

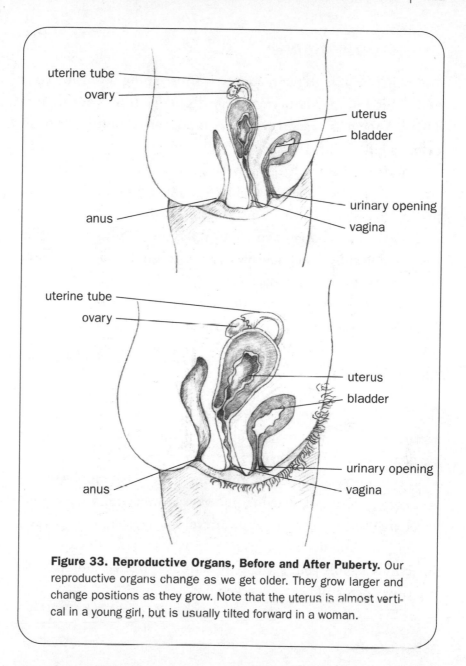

Figure 33. Reproductive Organs, Before and After Puberty. Our reproductive organs change as we get older. They grow larger and change positions as they grow. Note that the uterus is almost vertical in a young girl, but is usually tilted forward in a woman.

fact, in some women, it actually tilts backward. These positions are all perfectly normal.

VAGINAL DISCHARGE

You won't be able to see the growth spurt going on inside your body. But you may notice a watery discharge from your vagina. This is known as *vaginal discharge*. It appears about a year or so before a girl's first period.

Your vaginal discharge may be clear or white. As it dries on your underpants, it may be slightly yellow. It is perfectly normal, just another sign that you're growing up.

Vaginal discharge is the body's way of keeping the vagina clean and healthy. You know how your skin on the outside of your body is always shedding dead cells? Well, the walls of the vagina do the same. During puberty, the vagina sheds cells more quickly. Your body produces small amounts of fluid to wash these cells away. Vaginal discharge is a mixture of dead cells and the fluids that wash these cells away.

You may have more discharge on some days than on others. The color and texture may also change. At times, the discharge is clear and slippery. At other times, it's white and either creamy or thick and pasty. These changes are perfectly normal.

Infection can cause abnormal discharge. These problems are not common in girls starting puberty. However, if your vaginal discharge turns green or yellow, develops a strong odor, causes itching or redness, or is unusually heavy, see your doctor. Most infections in girls your age are not serious if treated promptly. So see your doctor and get it checked out.

HORMONES

Hormones cause the growth spurt in your reproductive organs. Hormones cause your vaginal discharge. In fact, hormones play a

---

hormones (HOR-moans)

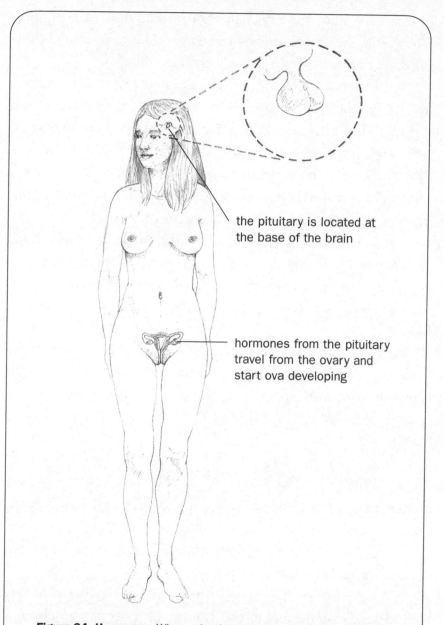

the pituitary is located at the base of the brain

hormones from the pituitary travel from the ovary and start ova developing

Figure 34. Hormones. When stimulated by hormones from the pituitary, the ovaries make increased amounts of the female hormone estrogen. Estrogen travels throughout a girl's body, causing many changes, including the swelling of the breasts and development of fat tissue around the hips.

role in almost all puberty changes. Breasts, pubic hair, pimples, body odor, the growth spurt—you name it! Hormones are behind all these changes. So what exactly are hormones?

Hormones are chemicals. They're made in certain parts of the body. They travel through the bloodstream to various body organs. They carry messages to tell these organs how to develop and work properly. Your body makes many different hormones. We'll talk only about the ones that cause puberty changes and direct the menstrual cycle. These hormones are made in the *pituitary gland* at the base of the brain and in the ovaries.

Puberty starts in your head, in the pituitary gland. Long before you notice any outward signs of puberty, this gland begins making a hormone that travels through the bloodstream to your ovaries. It causes your ovaries to make another hormone called *estrogen.*

Estrogen travels throughout the body. It causes many of the changes you notice as puberty starts. For example, estrogen causes fat pads to develop around your hips. It also causes your breasts to grow and develop. (See Figure 34.)

Estrogen and the Menstrual Cycle

Estrogen isn't just a puberty thing. It's a hormone that affects you not just during puberty, but for much of your life. For example, after a girl begins having periods, estrogen helps control the menstrual cycle. Here's how it works.

At the beginning of each menstrual cycle, the pituitary gland sends a hormone to the ovaries. This hormone delivers a message to the ova stored there. There are thousands of ova

pituitary (pu-TWO-uh-terr-ee)
estrogen (ES-tro-jen)

stored in each ovary. Each ovum lies inside its own tiny sac. The ova stored in a young girl's ovaries are not fully mature. They cannot ripen on their own. They must wait for the hormone from the pituitary. At the start of each menstrual cycle, the pituitary hormone reaches the ovary and causes about twenty ova to grow and develop.

As the ova develop, cells in the walls of the sacs that hold them make more and more estrogen. As a result, the level of estrogen in the bloodstream rises. This causes changes in the uterus. New blood vessels develop in the uterine lining. The lining quickly grows thicker—five times thicker, in fact! (If a woman becomes pregnant, this lining will help nourish the baby growing inside her.)

Ovulation

Meanwhile, back at the ovary, one of the developing ova grows much larger than the rest. It also makes much more estrogen than the others. This is the ovum that will be released during ovulation. Normally only one ovum is released when a woman

---

OVULATION PAIN

Most of us don't feel a thing when the bubble on the ovary bursts open, releasing its ovum. We're not even aware of it happening, but some women do have pain around the time of ovulation. This pain is called *Mittelschmerz*. (Don't even bother trying to pronounce this German word!) It's usually felt as a mild cramping pain on one side of the lower tummy, which usually lasts, at most, a few hours. For some women, though, the pain may last a day or two.

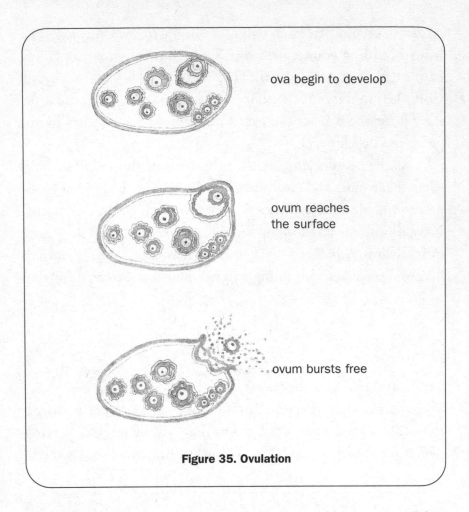

ova begin to develop

ovum reaches
the surface

ovum bursts free

Figure 35. Ovulation

ovulates. It's not clear how or why one particular ovum is "chosen" to mature fully, but, however this happens, other ova stop growing and shrink away.

The chosen ovum, nestled inside its own sac, grows so large that it presses against the outer wall of the ovary. It presses so hard that it forms a tiny bubble on the ovary's surface.

At this point, the level of estrogen reaches its peak. This high level of estrogen sends a message back to the pituitary. In

---

ovulates (OV-you-lates)

response, the pituitary produces a spurt of another hormone. Like the hormone that starts ova developing, this hormone also travels to the ovary. It causes the bubble on the ovary's surface to burst open and release the ovum. As we've said, this release of the mature ovum from the ovary is called ovulation. (See Figure 35.)

Fertilization

As the ovum pops off the ovary, the ends of the nearer uterine tube reach out like fingers. They sweep the ovum into the tube. The tube is lined with tiny hairs that wave back and forth. Slowly, over the next several days, they help move the ovum through the tube, toward the uterus.

The ovum may meet a male's sperm inside the tube. (If you recall from Chapter 1, a male may ejaculate sperm into his partner's vagina during sex. Some of the sperm may then swim into her uterus, and up into her tubes.)

If a couple has sex around the time of ovulation, there's a good chance the ovum will meet sperm in the tube. If so, one of the sperm may enter the ovum. This joining of the ovum and sperm is called fertilization. From the fertilized ovum, a baby can grow.

The ovum can only be fertilized in the first twenty-four hours after leaving the ovary, but sperm can stay alive in a woman's body for up to five days. So, sperm from sex that took place days before ovulation could "hang out" in the woman's body. When the ripe ovum enters the tube, the sperm could already be there, waiting for a chance to fertilize it. This means a woman can get pregnant if she has sex *at any time in the five days before ovulation or in the twenty-four hours after ovulation*. There is also a small chance of getting pregnant from having sex more than five days *before* or more than one day *after* ovulation.

Fertilized or not, the ovum continues to travel toward the uterus. It arrives in the uterus five to seven days after leaving the ovary. (See Figure 36.)

Meanwhile, back on the surface of the ovary, the remains of the bubble that once held the ripe ovum begin making still another hormone. This hormone is called *progesterone*. It causes the uterine lining to produce special fluids. These fluids help nourish a fertilized ovum in the early stages of pregnancy. By the time the ovum arrives in the uterus, the lining is very thick. If fertilized, the ovum plants itself in the lining within a few days. This sends a message to the ovary, which causes the remains of the burst bubble to continue making hormones. These hormones cause the uterine lining to remain thick, so that it can nourish the implanted ovum. Over the next nine months, the fertilized ovum grows into a baby.

Menstruation

If the ovum isn't fertilized, it doesn't plant itself in the uterine lining. Instead, it simply dissolves. Therefore, no message is sent to the ovary, and the remains of the burst bubble stop making progesterone.

When the progesterone level in the bloodstream drops, the lining of the uterus breaks down. Spongy tissues slide off the walls of the uterus. The tissues break down and liquefy. This liquid, along with blood from the lining, collects in the bottom of the uterus. (You can look back at Figure 11 in Chapter 1, on page 25.) From there, the blood and tissues trickle into the vagina and out the vaginal opening. This blood and tissue is called the menstrual flow. It usually continues for two to seven days before stopping. As we've said, these days of bleeding are called menstruation, or the menstrual period.

---

progesterone (pro-JES-ter-own)

MENOPAUSE

The menstrual cycles do not go on forever. When a woman reaches a certain age, usually between forty-five and fifty-five, her menstrual cycles stop. Her ovaries stop producing a ripe egg each month. She no longer has her monthly period, and she is no longer able to have a baby.

We have a special name for the time in a girl's life when she begins menstruating and ovulating. We call it *puberty*. We also have a name for the time in a woman's life when she stops menstruating and ovulating. It's called *menopause*.

THE MENSTRUAL CYCLE

It is the drop in the ovary's output of hormones that causes the uterine lining to break down and menstruation to begin. This drop has another effect, too. Once the hormones drop below a certain level, the pituitary kicks into action again. It again sends a hormone to the ovary, causing another group of twenty or so ova to begin developing. As the ova develop, they begin making larger and larger amounts of estrogen. And once again, the rising levels of estrogen cause the uterine lining to start growing thick. When the estrogen level peaks, another ripe ovum is released from the ovary. If it is not fertilized, the lining again breaks down and another period begins.

The menstrual cycle has been set in motion once again. The whole cycle repeats itself over and over again. Each repeated cycle is called one *menstrual cycle*. (See Figure 36.)

---

menopause (MEN-o-paws)

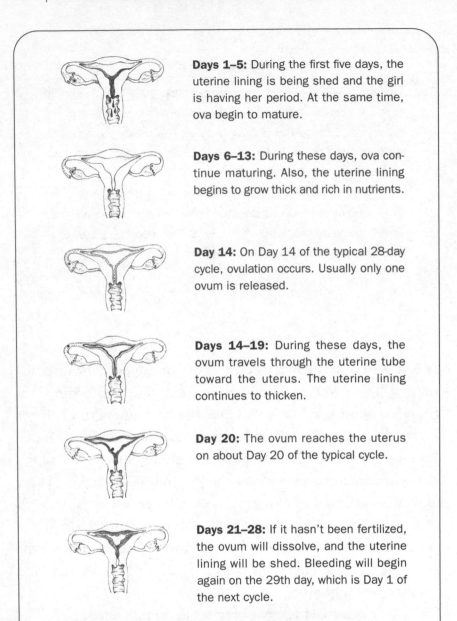

Days 1–5: During the first five days, the uterine lining is being shed and the girl is having her period. At the same time, ova begin to mature.

Days 6–13: During these days, ova continue maturing. Also, the uterine lining begins to grow thick and rich in nutrients.

Day 14: On Day 14 of the typical 28-day cycle, ovulation occurs. Usually only one ovum is released.

Days 14–19: During these days, the ovum travels through the uterine tube toward the uterus. The uterine lining continues to thicken.

Day 20: The ovum reaches the uterus on about Day 20 of the typical cycle.

Days 21–28: If it hasn't been fertilized, the ovum will dissolve, and the uterine lining will be shed. Bleeding will begin again on the 29th day, which is Day 1 of the next cycle.

Figure 36. A Typical Menstrual Cycle. A typical menstrual cycle lasts twenty-eight days. However, the length of a menstrual cycle may be quite a bit longer or shorter than twenty-eight days. Young girls who have just started menstruating are especially likely to have irregular menstrual cycles.

Length of the Cycle

The menstrual cycle begins with your period. The first day of your period is Day 1 of the menstrual cycle. The cycle continues with Day 2, Day 3, and so on, until the next menstrual period starts. The day the next period starts is Day 1 of that next menstrual cycle. One complete cycle runs from the first day of one period to the first day of the next period.

The length of the cycle is the number of days between periods. (See Figure 36.) The cycle length varies from woman to woman. It also varies in a single woman from one cycle to the next. In adult women, a menstrual cycle is usually somewhere between twenty-one and thirty-five days long. The average is about twenty-eight days, but there are very few women who actually have their periods every twenty-eight days, year in and year out.

One month a woman's cycle might last twenty-seven days. The next cycle might last twenty-nine days. The cycle after that might be thirty days long. Each of us has her own pattern. Some of us are more regular than others. In general, menstrual cycles tend to be most regular for women between the ages of twenty and forty. This isn't always the case, as one woman explains.

> I was very regular when I was younger. I could set my watch by it—once every twenty-six days. Then, when I turned thirty, I got real irregular—once every twenty-two days, once every twenty-six, once every thirty. Now I'm more regular again.
>
> —TRICIA, AGE 37

Doctors aren't always able to tell us why some women are regular and others aren't or why our patterns may change. We do know that traveling, emotional ups and downs, stress, and illness can affect the length of the cycle. Also, women who spend a lot of time with each other sometimes have cycles of the same length and get their periods around the same time. One woman told us:

> I've always menstruated about the same time as the other women I'm around. When I lived at home, my sisters and I always had our periods together. . . . When I went away to college, I found that my periods changed. I started menstruating around the middle of the month, same as my roommates.
>
> —TERRY, AGE 24

Irregular Cycles in Young Women

Young women who have just started having their periods are likely to be irregular. It takes a while for their bodies to get used to menstruating and ovulating. In fact, young girls often have cycles in which they menstruate but do not ovulate.

It often takes two or three years before a girl has a regular pattern of ovulation and menstruation. The first few periods are especially likely to be irregular. However, even when they're irregular, the cycles are usually between twenty-one to forty-four days long.

In the past, doctors didn't worry too much if a young girl had cycles longer or shorter than this. They thought it was just part of the irregular cycles young women are known to have. However, many doctors have changed their thinking on this. They feel a girl should be checked by a doctor if she repeatedly has cycles shorter than twenty-one days or longer than forty-four days. Having longer or shorter cycles than usual doesn't always mean a girl has a medical problem, but because she *might* have a problem, many doctors feel she should be checked.

Length of Period

Your period may last anywhere from two to seven days. The average is about five days. The length of your period may vary from one cycle to the next. For example, one cycle you may bleed for three days and the next cycle for six days. After the time between periods becomes more regular, the length of your periods usually becomes more regular, too. When a woman approaches menopause, the length of her periods may again start to vary more from one period to the next.

At any time of life, bleeding for more than seven days is considered abnormal. If your periods consistently last more than seven days, see your doctor. This usually isn't the sign of a serious problem, but long periods, especially if there's heavy bleeding, can cause anemia and a tired-out feeling, so get it checked out.

Amount and Pattern of Menstrual Flow

Although it may seem as if a lot of blood comes out when you have your period, it isn't really that much. From the beginning to the end of your period the menstrual flow usually totals about one-quarter to one-third cup.

Some months your period may be heavier than others. This is quite normal, but sometimes the bleeding can be too heavy. See a doctor if you are soaking through a pad or tampon every hour for an entire day. (Pads and tampons are used to absorb the menstrual flow. See Chapter 7.) By the way, we mean literally soaking through, so the pad or tampon is filled with blood.

In a grown woman, the flow is usually heaviest on the first two or three days of her period. For the first two to three years after a girl begins to menstruate, she may have more erratic bleeding patterns. The pattern may vary from cycle to cycle.

DOUCHING

Douching flushes out the vagina with either plain water or water mixed with vinegar or a douche powder. These days douches often come in prefilled plastic bottles. The bottle has a nozzle on one end. The woman lies in an empty tub and inserts the nozzle into the vagina. She then squeezes the bottle. This forces the liquid into the vagina, flushing it out.

Douching really isn't a good idea. It's not necessary because, as you may recall from earlier in this chapter, fluids from the cervix and vaginal walls rinse your vagina and keep it clean naturally. These fluids help prevent infection. Douching can even be harmful because it can change the natural chemical balance in your vagina and lead to infections. There's also the chance of pushing infection up into the uterus. For all these reasons, girls should not douche.

Clots and the Color of the Flow

The menstrual flow may have thick clumps of blood called clots. You are more likely to notice clots if you've been sitting or lying down for a while and then change position. The clots form when the blood "pools" in the top of the vagina while you are sitting or lying down. You're most likely to have clots in the morning when you first get up. As long as the amount of flow is normal, clots aren't anything to worry about.

The menstrual flow may be pink, bright red, dark red, brown, or somewhere in between. All these colors are normal. The color may also vary from one period to the next or even from day to day during your period. Again, this is perfectly normal.

---

douching (DOOSH-ing)

Blood tends to turn brown when it comes in contact with air. If your menstrual flow has been slow in moving out of your body, it may take on a brownish color. It is especially likely to be brownish toward the end of your period.

Missed Periods

Sometimes you may miss a period or stop having periods altogether. Among women who have had sex, the most common cause of missed periods is pregnancy. So if you have had sex and you miss a period, see a doctor or go to a clinic right away. You may be pregnant.

There are other reasons why you might miss a period. Missed periods are especially common among young women who've just started menstruating. Even women who have been menstruating regularly for a number of years sometimes skip a period.

It's normal to miss an occasional period, but if you've been having periods regularly and then miss periods, that may be a sign that something is wrong. If you're not sexually active and can't be pregnant, you should be checked out by a doctor if you miss three periods in a row. Some doctors would recommend a girl be checked if she's missed two periods in a row.

Spotting

Spotting between periods may be literally just a spot, or a day or two of very light bleeding. It's not unusual to have some spotting for a day or two around the time of ovulation. You can figure out if your bleeding is related to ovulation. Keep track of your menstrual cycles. Note the dates when spotting occurs and the dates your periods begin. Spotting that happens about two weeks before your period starts is probably related to ovulation. This type of spotting isn't anything to worry about. If the spotting occurs at other times and continues for more than three cycles, see your doctor.

Just Guidelines

In the last pages, we've tried to give you an idea of what's normal and what's not when it comes to the menstrual cycle and the menstrual period. Remember, though, the information in this chapter is just a guideline. If you feel something about your menstrual cycle isn't right, see your doctor. If you do have a problem, you'll have caught it that much earlier. If you don't, then you can stop worrying.

OTHER MENSTRUAL CHANGES

Women may notice changes in their bodies or in their emotions during certain times in their menstrual cycle. One woman I know gets very energetic during her period. She often gets into fits of housecleaning (which is nice because, most of the time, she's not too interested in housework). In the week to ten days before their period starts, some women's breasts get lumpy, swollen, and tender. Another woman told me about what she called the "lead vagina." On the first couple of days of her period her vagina and vulva feel heavy, as though "they're made of lead." Quite a few women have strong sexual feelings when they're about to ovulate.

Most girls and women we talked to noticed some emotional or physical changes related to their menstrual cycle. Most of these changes happen during their periods or in the week or so before their periods. These are some changes you may experience before or during your period:

extra energy
lack of energy or a tired, dragged-out feeling
sudden shifts in moods
tension or anxiety
depression
feelings of well-being
bursts of creativity
craving for sweets
pimples, acne, or other skin problems
a particularly clear and rosy glow to the skin
heightened sexual feelings
headaches
vision disturbances
diarrhea
constipation
swelling of the ankles, wrists, hands, or feet
swelling and tenderness of the breasts
swelling of the abdomen
bloated feeling
temporary weight gain (usually three to five pounds)
decreased ability to concentrate
increased ability to concentrate
increased appetite
increased thirst
cramps
increased need to urinate
urinary infections
change in vaginal discharge
nausea
runny nose
sores in the mouth
backache

In some women, these changes are very noticeable. In others, they are hardly noticeable at all. And some women don't notice any of these changes.

PREMENSTRUAL SYNDROME

If a woman has one or more of the negative changes listed above during the seven to ten days before her menstrual period, she may have premenstrual syndrome, or *PMS*. No one is sure what causes PMS. Some doctors think that vitamin and nutritional deficiencies cause PMS. Others think it's due to a hormone imbalance.

Mild forms of PMS are quite widespread. Many of us experience PMS symptoms at some time in our lives. A bloated feeling, pimples, or swelling of the breasts are some of the most common PMS symptoms.

If you have mild PMS symptoms, there are some things you can try. You can cut out sugar, coffee, and chocolate from your diet. Eat balanced meals with foods rich in vitamin B6 and magnesium (green vegetables, whole grains, nuts, and seeds). Take a vitamin supplement that includes the B-complex vitamins. Some doctors use hormones to treat PMS, but others are not sure that hormone treatments really work.

If you think you have PMS, you should see a doctor who knows about PMS.

KEEPING TRACK OF YOUR MENSTRUAL CYCLE

It's a good idea to keep a record of your menstrual cycles. This way you can know what changes, like spotting at the time of ovulation, happen during your menstrual cycle. You'll also learn how your own pattern works and about when to expect your next period. (Remember, though, you may not be very regular at first.)

You'll need a calendar. On the first day of your period mark an *x* on your calendar. Then mark an x for each day the bleeding continues. When your next period starts, mark an x again. You can count the number of days between your periods. That way you'll begin to get an idea of how long your menstrual cycle usually lasts. (See Figure 37.)

You might also want to make a note of cramps, ovulation pain, or any other menstrual changes you may notice. For instance, you may find that you have a craving for sweets. Or you may feel tense and cranky, or your breasts may be tender. Note these events on your calendar. In this way, you can learn if certain changes occur at the same time during each menstrual cycle.

Once you begin to ovulate and menstruate in a regular cycle, you may also notice that your vaginal discharge changes over the course of your menstrual cycle.

Vaginal discharge has a different pattern in different women. Also, for some women these changes are more noticeable than in other women. Still, there is a general pattern for vaginal discharge that goes something like this:

On the days immediately following a woman's menstrual period, there is usually less vaginal discharge. The vagina and vaginal lips are apt to feel rather dry. A few days later, the amount of vaginal discharge increases. The vagina and vaginal lips are noticeably wetter. The discharge on these days may be clear, white, or yellowish. It may be thin and watery or rather thick and sticky.

Around the time of ovulation the amount of discharge increases still more. This discharge tends to be clear and quite slippery. It can stretch into long, shimmery strands. This type of mucus is called *fertile mucus* because it appears at the time of the

---

fertile mucus (FUR-tull MEW-kuss)

S	M	T	W	T	F	S
		1	2	3	4	5
6	7	8	✗9	✗10	✗11	✗12
✗13	✗14	15	16	17	18	19
20	21	22	23	24	25	26
27	28	29	30			

S	M	T	W	T	F	S
				1	2	3
4	5	6	7	✗8	✗9	✗10
✗11	✗12	13	14	15	16	17
18	19	20	21	22	23	24
25	26	27	28	29	30	31

Figure 37. Recording Your Periods. To keep track of your periods, use a calendar like this. This girl had her first day of bleeding on the ninth and she continued to bleed for 5 more days, so she marked these days with x's. The next cycle began on the eighth of the following month and her period lasted 5 days, which are marked with x's. By counting the number of days between x's (23 days for this girl), and adding the number of days of the first period (6 days for this girl), you can determine the length of your menstrual cycle. Since 23 plus 6 equals 29, this girl's cycle was 29 days long.

month when a woman is most fertile, or most likely to get pregnant. Fertile mucus has a chemical makeup that actually helps sperm on their journey to the ovum and thereby increases a woman's chances of getting pregnant.

Within one to three or more days after ovulation, the fertile mucus disappears. Some women don't have much discharge from this point until their next period. Their vagina and vaginal lips again feel rather dry. Other women continue to have some discharge and a feeling of wetness, but the mucus is quite different from the fertile mucus. It tends to be rather sticky. Still other women alternate between dry and wet days.

You may want to keep track of the changes in your vaginal discharge. You can record these changes on your calendar as well.

All this helps you learn about your body's own special patterns.

In this chapter we talked about the things that happen to you during your menstrual cycle, as well as what's normal when you have your period. In the next chapter we'll get into all kinds of practical details about periods, including the choices you have for menstrual protection.

7.
ALL
ABOUT HAVING
PERIODS

When will I get my first period?

Girls often ask this question. We wish we had an answer. We don't. No one can tell ahead of time when a girl's first period will come, but this chapter has some info to help you make an educated guess. In this chapter, we'll also give you some advice about what to do if you get your period at school. You'll hear what the girls and women in our classes and workshops had to say about their first periods.

This chapter isn't just for girls who haven't started to menstruate yet. There's also lots of information for girls who have already started. In this chapter, we talk about tampons and pads, as well as some of the new products on the market, and the debate over the safety of some of these products. You'll also learn about cramps and how to cope with them.

GETTING YOUR FIRST PERIOD

The average age of starting to menstruate varies a bit between different racial and ethnic groups. For example, among white girls in this country, the average age for the first period is twelve years and ten and a half months. Among African-American girls, it's twelve years and two months. Other racial and ethnic groups in this country have not been studied, but, in all groups, the average age is probably between the twelfth and thirteenth birthday.

Remember, though, we're not all average. (You're probably sick of our telling you this, but it's true.) Like other puberty changes, the first period happens within a wide range of ages. A girl may get her first period any time between the ages of nine and fifteen and a half.

There are even some perfectly healthy, normal girls who start earlier or later than this. Still, girls who start having periods before the age of nine should see a doctor. Likewise, girls who haven't had a period by the age of fifteen and a half should see a doctor. Although not starting within these age ranges may not mean anything at all, it could be the sign of a medical problem that needs treatment. So see a doctor and get checked out.

Breast Stage and Your First Period

Your stage of breast development is a much better clue to when you can expect your first period than your age. Most girls have their first period either toward the end of Breast Stage 3 or early in Breast Stage 4. This isn't a hard-and-fast rule. Although it is rare, a girl may start her period when she's only in Stage 2. Also, girls sometimes don't start their periods until Stage 5. Still, if you've been in Breast Stage 3 for a while or have just entered Stage 4, your first period is probably not too far off.

Family Background and Your First Period

Another clue: Daughters often have their first period around the same age their mothers had theirs. Younger sisters also tend to start within a month or two of when their older sisters started. Again, these are not hard-and-fast rules, but they hold true in many cases. It's worth finding out when your mom and any older sisters got their first period.

In Chapter 3, you learned that girls seem to be starting puberty earlier than in the past. Today's girls develop pubic hair and breasts at younger ages than girls did ten or twenty years ago. Are they also getting their period earlier?

In general, the answer seems to be "no." Among white girls in the United States, the average age for starting periods is the same today as it was forty years ago. Among African-American girls, the average age hasn't changed by more than a few months, if it's changed at all. (We don't know for sure. Only recently have there been good studies of African-American girls.)

Getting It at School

You could get your first period anytime—night or day. You could get it anywhere—at home or wherever. There's no way of knowing. "What'll I do if it happens when I'm at school?" the girls in our classes and workshops want to know. Luckily, there are usually lots of experts (girls who've already started to menstruate) with helpful advice. They share their stories with the other girls. Here's what one girl had to say:

> I got my first period during history class. I wasn't sure if it was happening, but I sort of knew. So I raised my hand and said I had to go to the bathroom. Sure enough, there was

blood on my underpants. I luckily had my purse with some change in it, so I got a sanitary napkin out of the machine and pinned it to my underpants and just went back to class.

—TONI, AGE 13

As she said, this girl was lucky. There was a sanitary napkin machine in the girl's room and she had some change with her. (A sanitary napkin is a menstrual pad. Pads are worn inside your panties to absorb—soak up—the menstrual flow.) Another girl wasn't so lucky, but things still worked out fine for her.

I got my period at school, too. I kinda knew right away what it was. I went to the bathroom to check. There weren't any napkins in the machine. I just wadded up some toilet paper and went to the nurse's office. She was real nice and gave me a clean pair of underpants and a napkin.

—ROSE, AGE 13

Many girls used tissues or toilet paper to line their panties until they could get a pad. Some girls got a pad from a woman at school. Sometimes it was the school nurse or a gym teacher. Other times it was another teacher or a secretary in the school office. If their underpants were bloody, sometimes the nurse or someone else had a spare pair. Others just ignored the blood or rinsed their pants out with cold water. Some girls called their moms, who brought clean pants and pads to school. One girl told how she prepared for her first period.

I knew I was getting old enough. At the beginning of seventh grade, I put a sanitary napkin in my purse—in those special carrying cases they give you. I just kept it there so I'd be ready. The school I was going to didn't have a school nurse.

The machines were always broken or empty. I didn't want to have to go into the office and say I was having my period. There were always a lot of people in there. I would have been so embarrassed.

—SANDY, AGE 14

The classic menstrual horror story goes something like this. A girl's menstrual flow bleeds through her underwear and shows on her outer clothing. Meanwhile, she's totally clueless. She's walking around school (or some other public place) unaware of the big red spot on the back of her white skirt or white pants or white shorts.

If you notice, the girl is almost always wearing something white in these stories. It's never something black or blue or purple. And these stories are almost always told by somebody who knew somebody who knew somebody who it actually happened to. Once, though, we heard it firsthand.

SAYING YOU DID WHEN YOU DIDN'T

Your friends and classmates have all gotten their periods. Everyone . . . except you! Your friends are talking about their periods and suddenly everyone is looking at you. The spotlight is on you. It wouldn't be too surprising if you were to blurt out, "I got my period."

Should you feel terrible because you told a lie? We don't think so. Besides, it's not the kind of lie you'll have to live with forever. Sooner or later it *will* be true.

In the meantime, keep remembering you're special. Your period *will* come. Your body is doing exactly what's right for you. What's important is to feel good about yourself.

I had that napkin in my purse for almost a year. I thought I was so smart—being ready and all. Then I'm walking down the hall one day and my girlfriend says, "Hey, you got blood on your skirt." I almost died. "Stand in back of me," I said. She walked down the hall kind of right behind me, so no one could see. I got my coat out of my locker and put it on and went to the office. I told the secretary I was sick and had to go home.

—HEATHER, AGE 13

We have no doubt that Heather was telling the truth, but things like this don't happen too often. Most girls notice a feeling of wetness before any blood soaks through their underpants and onto their clothes. Besides, most girls don't bleed enough right at first to have it show through on their clothes.

Think about it. How often have you seen a girl walking around in public with menstrual blood on her clothing? Not too often, we bet. Maybe never. It just doesn't happen that often.

If you're worried about getting your period, talk it over with your mom, older sister, or another woman you trust. She might have some helpful hints. Just talking about your worries can help a lot.

Girls often want to know what it feels like to get your first period. You'll hear many different answers in the quotes from girls and women in the next few pages. Many girls notice a feeling of wetness or have a stomach ache or cramps when they get their first period. Others don't feel anything. They discover they've started to menstruate only when they notice some blood on their underwear or pajamas.

More First Period Stories

I was visiting with my grandmother at her house. We were talking and playing games one afternoon. I noticed that my underpants were feeling more and more wet. I also felt like I had a bit of a stomach ache. After about an hour, the wetness seemed to increase and I went to the bathroom to investigate. There was a small blood stain on my underpants. The "wet" and "achy stomach" feelings were my only warning. There were no painful cramps.

—CHERRY, AGE 30

I thought I'd bleed a lot. I worried a lot about it. I thought it would be like a flood, like this big glop of blood was gonna plop on the floor. It was more like a stain . . . a few drops . . . I didn't have a clue. I just went to the bathroom. That's when I saw the stain.

—TINA, AGE 14

I got mine in second-period class. I happened to go to the bathroom. I noticed some little brownish spots on my underwear. I went back to class and got my best friend and described it to her. She said it was my period, and we were both really excited.

—LAURA, AGE 36

Many girls—especially those who started later than their friends—felt relieved when they finally got their period.

When I first started my period, I was sixteen. I was in gym class changing back into school clothes. I used a tampon and stayed in school. When I got home I told my mom. I felt very relieved because I thought there was something wrong with my body. It was embarrassing because all my friends and my sister started theirs early. However, overall, I felt different about me. I felt, "Now I'm normal."

—AMY, AGE 18

I was actually very disturbed about not having my period. My friends had all started at twelve. Not only that, but I had almost no breasts. I had recently asked my mother if perhaps I was really a boy. She assured me that I was quite normal. I didn't really believe her. . . . Finally, finally, I got my period!

—YOLANDA, AGE 36

I still didn't have my period and I was worried. I even made my mom take me to the doctor. The very next week I started my period. I was really relieved, but I sorta wished I hadn't wasted my time at the doctor.

—SALLY, AGE 35

I had my first period. . . . I felt very glad because I felt like I was finally a woman. All my friends had it earlier. My sister got it younger, too. When I finally got it, I told my mom. . . . I felt— before I had my period—that there was something wrong with me. My friends were getting it at twelve or thirteen. I felt like something was missing in me. I spoke to my mother about it. She said, "We all get it at different times." She was supportive.

—EVA, AGE 26

Some girls were scared at first. Many were embarrassed when they got their first period or worried that other people could tell.

I was twelve. I was asleep and woke up, had to go to the bathroom. I was kind of dripping on the way. It was a very scary experience. My mom had told me about it, but I wasn't interested. I had forgotten all about it by the time it happened. I didn't say anything. That night I washed my sheets. I had to wash the rug. I was devastated. I think it was about two days later when I told my mom.

Until that point, I was ashamed because I thought I was too young to have gotten it. My mom, however, was very excited, told my dad right away, and then proceeded to tell the rest of my family during dinner.

—MARINA, AGE 16

I got my period when I was ten. I was taking my swimming lesson. I knew what was happening, but it was embarrassing. My mom told Grandma when we got home, and I was embarrassed . . . about the whole experience. I felt shocked, surprised, and like I was growing up.

—SHANA, AGE 15

My birthday is June 20, 1937. My period began on May 5, 1949. . . . I remember the date because Liz Taylor was getting married for the first time that day, to Nicky Hilton. I was an avid reader of movie magazines by then.

I was spending the weekend at my pal Dixie's house in the officers' quarters of the naval base. We went swimming at the base pool, and that's where it started. Somehow I made it to the dressing room, but I can still remember looking around at all the sailors and wondering if they knew. It's a sensitive memory for me.

When I got home, mother showed me how to use a Kotex [pad]. It surprised me. I had seen them in her bathroom. I had even used one once for a bandage, but it was the first time she mentioned the word "menstruation" to me. Afterward, I got on my bike and rode over to my friend Pam's to tell her the big news.

—FRANCINE, AGE 70

Emotional reactions to starting to menstruate were as varied as the girls and women we talked to. Many described themselves as "freaked out." Others were indifferent or at least not "majorly shocked."

I was fourteen and I was at school. I felt wet, went to the bathroom, and freaked out. "Oh, it's my thing!" Totally embarrassed, panicked, I wanted to find my sister, the only person I wanted to deal with on the planet. I took toilet paper and wadded it up. Then I went back to study hall and acted like everything was all right. After study hall, I found my sister and I can't remember, but everything got okay.

—AMANDA, AGE 50

I was twelve. I got it in school. When I went to the bathroom, I had a feeling I was getting it because a lot of my friends were getting it. I went to the bathroom, and, yes, there was blood on my underwear. I wadded up a big wad of toilet paper. I had about an hour left in school. I figured I'd just stay and go home on the bus like normal. When I got home, I called my mom at work to tell her. I told her she had to bring some Kotex [pads] home. I just took it with indifference.

—LEONA, AGE 15

I started my period when I was eleven. . . . I wasn't ready with any pads or tampons or anything. It was during the summer between sixth and seventh grade. I was at home. I went to my mom afterward. My mom said (not much) simply, "We gotta go out and get some pads." I felt like I was growing up. I'm becoming a woman. I wasn't majorly shocked.

—TOYA, AGE 16

I didn't feel ashamed or embarrassed about my body. Overall, it was a positive experience. Although I had a hard time—I felt bad cramps and had heavy bleeding. After I realized it wasn't so hard, I found myself wondering why I had been so anxious about getting it.

—SHIRLEE, AGE 36

Most of the "first period" stories we've heard were basically positive ones. The only negative stories we heard were from girls whose mothers had not prepared them for their first period.

I was eleven when I got my period. I had gone to the bathroom and found blood streaming out of me. I went crazy. I thought I was dying. I panicked and started screaming. I ran out of the bathroom into the living room and everyone there laughed at me. No one had ever told me a thing about it and then they laughed at my reaction. I felt terrified and stupid.

—JOAN, AGE 46

I was eleven and one half. I was at home and my stomach hurt. It felt like number two or a diarrhea cramp. I went to the bathroom. When I got on the toilet, I found that brownish red stuff was coming out of me. In my sixth-grade class they had just shown films about menstruation, so I knew what it was. My mom had not talked to me about it. I was raised in a very strict Christian home. I ran out of the bathroom excited to tell Mom, "I am a woman now!"

When I happily told her what had happened, she frowned and told me where the maxi pads were in the bathroom. She seemed like she didn't want me to have it. Within one week, my parents took me to a doctor and asked him to put me on birth control. (I was still a virgin.) This embarrassed me and I was humiliated that I had gotten my period. I called my best friend. When I told her, she was very happy and congratulated me, and so did her mother. At this point I was very confused and did not know how to act, so I just kept quiet and didn't tell anyone else.

—CHRISTINA, AGE 30

Christina's story was the only one we heard where the mom wasn't as happy and excited as the daughter about the big news. In fact, sometimes the parents seemed more excited than the girls themselves. On the whole, the mothers and daughters we talked to were very happy and excited about getting their period.

I was very excited when it happened. I thought, "Well, now maybe I will get big boobs!"

—MAXINE, AGE 12

I finally got my period when I was sixteen years old. I was at Bonnie and Betty's house—twins who were my very close friends, along with the two Nancys and Judy. This was our group. We did everything together. I went to the bathroom and, lo and behold, there was blood. . . . I told all the girls. They all cheered. They were as excited as I was.

—NAOMI, AGE 25

Telling Your Parents

Getting your period is one thing. Telling your parents is another. At least, it is for some girls. Here's what three readers who wrote to us had to say:

My mom never talked to me about periods or anything. I'm scared to think about telling her when I get mine.

Help! I got my period again (three times so far). I haven't even told my mom that I started periods yet.

My mom died when I was little. I'm too embarrassed to talk to my dad. I don't know what I'll do when my period comes.

Does any of this sound familiar to you? If so, we hope the advice below will help you break the big news.

If you've already started your period, how about the direct approach? Just say, "Guess what, I got my period!"

If that's too direct, how about this? You buy a "congratulations" card at the store. Get one that doesn't say exactly what the congrats are for. Then write in something like, "Congrats, you are now the parent of a menstruating daughter."

If it's easier to tell your mom than your dad, that's fine. A lot of girls feel that way. Not all girls have a mom living in their home, though. If you live with just your dad, you could ask a female relative or close family friend to help you tell your dad. But don't write your dad off just because he's a man. Guys know about these things, too. The first time a single-parent father and his daughter signed up for our puberty workshop, some of the mothers were worried about having him there, but he was the hit of the workshop. After that, more and more fathers started showing up at workshops, and it's always great to have them.

If you haven't gotten your period yet and you think your parents may be uncomfortable talking about it with you, you've got time to prepare them for the big event. That way it will be much easier to tell them when you do get it. You could break the ice by bringing up the subject in a casual way. You might ask your mom how old she was when she got her first period, how she told her mom, or how she felt about getting it. You could ask your mom or dad if they had sex education classes in school or if they think girls are having periods earlier today than in the past.

Another way to get them talking is to ask for their help in inventing a puberty rite. Female puberty rites are ceremonies to mark a girl's first menstrual period. They've existed in cultures all over the world and throughout human history. Some rites grew

---

IS IT ALL RIGHT TO . . . ?

There are lots of rumors about what you should and should not do during your periods. Girls ask us if it's all right to take a bath or shower, to wash their hair, to go horseback riding, to have sex, to drink cold drinks, and so forth. The answer to all these questions is "yes." If you can do it when you're not having your period, you can do it during your period.

Don't believe all the nonsense you hear. Neither cold food or drinks nor heavy exercise causes a heavier flow, longer periods, or cramps. And you should definitely shower or bathe during your period! Since blood can develop an odor after a while, a daily shower or bath is a must.

You can do anything you'd do at any other time of the month. Of course, if you're going swimming, you'll want to use a tampon, not a pad. (See pages 175–183.)

out of primitive, fearful beliefs about menstruation and were pretty horrible, but some were real celebrations. For example, in parts of India, the rite started with a big feast. It ended with the girl sitting on a throne, while her friends, neighbors, and relatives laid gifts at her feet!

It's unlikely that you'll be able to sell your parents on the throne-and-gifts-at-your-feet routine, but why not invent a modern puberty rite of your own? You might invent a special moonlight ceremony, have a slumber party with all your female friends, or be given a ring or special gift to be passed on to the next generation. It could be anything. One father we know promised to take his daughter on a trip of her choosing. When the big day came, off they went to Las Vegas! Whatever you plan, the simple fact that you've made plans will make it easier to tell your parents when you get your period.

MENSTRUAL PROTECTION

Over the ages, women have used everything from grass to sea sponges to folded rags to catch their menstrual flow. Today, we have lots of choices.

There are many different products on the market. They're called menstrual protection products. (Makes it sound like your period is going to attack you, doesn't it?) These products don't, as the name implies, protect you from your period. They protect your clothes from menstrual blood stains. It's a dumb term, but at least it's better than *feminine hygiene products*, which is the other name for this group of products.

Most women in this country use pads, tampons, or both during their periods. The soft material in these products absorbs the menstrual flow. The difference is in how they're worn. Tampons are inserted into the vagina. Pads are worn outside the body. There are over 150 different styles and brands of pads and tampons. There are also some entirely new products on the market. With so many choices, it can be hard to decide which product to use.

In the following pages we'll tell you about what's available. We'll fill you in on the nitty-gritty details of using these products. If you have access to the Internet, you can visit the websites of the different companies that make these products. (You'll find a list of websites in the Resource Section.) You might also get some helpful advice by asking your mom or another woman you trust what she uses and why.

Tampon Safety and TSS

TSS is short for *toxic shock syndrome*. It is a rare but very serious condition. It can affect people of any age and either sex. Most cases of TSS have been linked to the use of tampons. It's not that tampons carry germs. TSS is caused by common bacteria that live on the surface of the skin and in the vagina. Normally these bacteria don't cause any problem, but in a small number of women these bacteria have caused TSS. TSS can cause serious side effects and, in a small number of cases, death.

TSS usually starts with a sudden fever, vomiting, and diarrhea. Sometimes there is a headache, sore throat, or achy muscles. Within forty-eight hours the person may become very weak and groggy. A red rash that winds up peeling like sunburn may develop. When TSS is associated with tampon use, the symptoms may appear during the period or in the first few days after the period.

There are ways to reduce the risk of TSS. Since blood is a rich breeding ground for bacteria, leaving a tampon in too long

---

toxic (TOK-sick)

allows the bacteria to multiply. Women who use the super-absorbent kind of tampon usually change their tampons less often. This makes them more prone to infection. Use the less absorbent kind of tampons and change them every four to eight hours. (For more information read "Choosing the Right Absorbency" on page 178.)

Questions About Dioxin

Recently, there have been new questions about the safety of menstrual protection products. Some people are concerned about the possible presence of a chemical called *dioxin* in tampons and, to a lesser extent, in pads. Dioxin is a very toxic substance. Doctors think it may cause cancer. In small quantities it can enter our bodies in a number of different ways. Because it's very slow to leave the body, repeated exposures to dioxin keep building up its level in the body. As a result, any harmful effects from dioxin might take a long time to show up.

Several years ago, the Food and Drug Administration (FDA) asked tampon manufacturers to test their products for dioxin. The result showed either no detectable dioxin or dioxin at very low levels. Many people, including the FDA, believed that dioxin at these very low levels did not pose a health risk. However, no one knows just what level of dioxin is harmful in people. So the controversy continued, with some experts feeling that even the very low dioxin level found in tampons might pose a health risk.

At the time of the testing requested by the FDA, rayon and cotton fibers in tampons and pads were usually bleached using *chlorine*. This chlorine-based bleaching was a source of dioxin.

---

dioxin (deye-AHK-sin)
chlorine (KLOOR-een)

Now, however, as part of efforts to keep all dioxin out of the environment, no U.S. manufacturer of tampons uses rayon or cotton that has been bleached with chlorine. So today, according to the FDA, tampons are not contaminated with dioxin.

Pads

Pads are made from layers of soft, absorbent material. Most have a super-absorbent inner core to help keep blood from soaking through the pad. Pads attach to your underpants. The most popular type is held in place by sticky strips on the pad's underside. You just peel off the glossy paper and press the pad, sticky side down, onto your underpants. (See Figure 38.) Some pads also have "wings" that help to prevent leaks and hold the pad more firmly in place. (See Figure 39.) The wings fold over and also stick to the outside of your underpants by adhesive or Velcro.

There's also an older-style pad. This type attaches to your panties with safety pins or to a sanitary napkin belt. Most stores no longer carry this kind of pad, and the belts are even harder to find.

A Buyer's Guide to Pads

Maxi Pads, Thin Maxis, Ultra Thin Maxis, Thin Super Maxi Pads, Ultra Thin Long Maxis With Wings . . . Confused by these product names? If so, you aren't alone. Don't worry, though—we'll help you sort it out. It all boils down to four basics.

- SHAPE: Some pads are flat with straight sides. Others have an hourglass shape. Some curve rather than lie flat. There are also pads with side flaps called "wings," "tabs," or "plus." The flaps wrap around the sides of your panties and attach on the underside. Which is best? It's really a matter of personal choice.

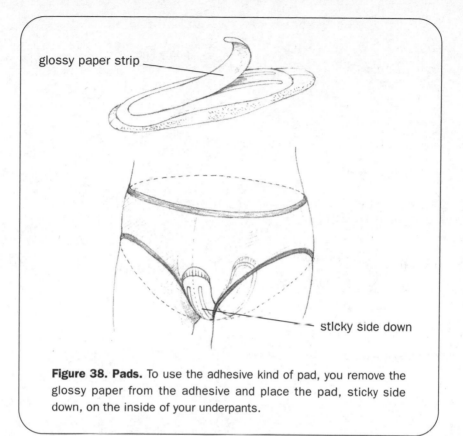

glossy paper strip

stIcky side down

Figure 38. Pads. To use the adhesive kind of pad, you remove the glossy paper from the adhesive and place the pad, sticky side down, on the inside of your underpants.

- WIDTH: Some companies make "slim," "slender," or "junior" pads for small-bodied women and girls. They're not as wide as other pads. If your pads bunch up or twist out of shape, try these narrow pads.

- LENGTH: Pads can "ride up" or slip back so that they wind up too far forward or too far back. The result: Blood winds up on panties instead of the pad. Sound familiar? If so, look for the words "long," "longer," or "extra length" on the box.

- THICKNESS: Most brands come in three thicknesses—regular, thin, and ultra thin. Some companies also make panty liners, which are the thinnest pads, or very thick overnight

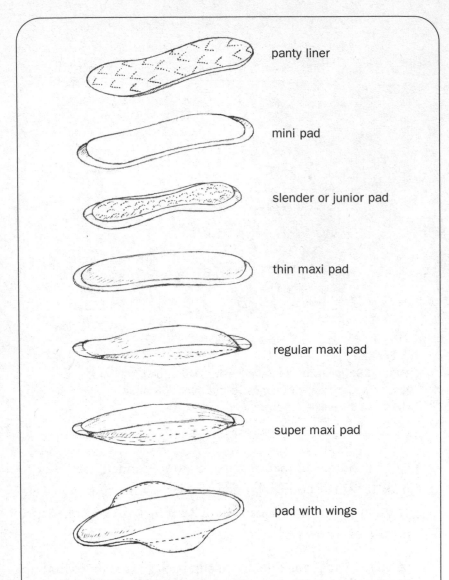

panty liner

mini pad

slender or junior pad

thin maxi pad

regular maxi pad

super maxi pad

pad with wings

Figure 39. Types of Pads. Some of the many different types of pads are shown in this figure. Panty liners are the thinnest and least absorbent. Mini pads are a little thicker than panty liners. Super maxi pads are the thickest and most absorbent of all. Slender or junior pads are designed especially for teens. They're shorter and slimmer than maxi pads. Pads with "wings" wrap around the sides of your panties.

pads. The panty liners aren't very absorbent. Even on your lightest days, they may not do the job. But some girls like to use them with a tampon as a backup in case of leaks.

Regular, thin, and even ultra thin pads can absorb quite a bit of fluid. In general, though, the ultra thins absorb more slowly than other pads. This can be a problem if you have a sudden rush of blood, which can happen when you cough, sneeze, move after sitting for a while, and at other times, too.

Using Pads

Wearing a pad may seem a bit strange at first. It may feel like you've got a rolled-up beach towel stuffed in your panties. You're sure everyone can tell. Really, though, it doesn't show. Check it out in the mirror. You'll see—the pad really isn't visible.

Pads are easy to use. (If you can walk and chew gum at the same time, you can definitely manage a pad.) There are only a couple of rules to remember.

- CHANGE YOUR PAD OFTEN: Even if your flow is light, change your pad every four to six hours during the day so that it won't smell. Menstrual blood itself is perfectly clean and odorless, but once it comes in contact with air, germs start to grow. They can cause an unpleasant odor. Change your pad often, and the odor won't have a chance to develop. You can wear a pad overnight. We recommend using pads overnight instead of tampons.

- DON'T FLUSH PADS DOWN THE TOILET: Pads can clog the plumbing. Even if the pad is biodegradable or flushable, it may clog older plumbing.

• WRAP USED PADS BEFORE DISPOSING OF THEM: No, not with ribbons and bows. Fold the pad in half and wrap it in tissue or toilet paper. Then toss it in the trash. Wrapping the pad cuts down on odor.

Reusable, 100% Cotton Pads

"Reusable pads—oh gross!" is a pretty typical reaction. But Glad Rags, one of the makers of these cloth pads, gives this response in a company booklet: Just envision your lifetime supply of used pads and tampons in landfills or washed up on a beach. Now that's gross!

Each year, women in the United States use over 12 billion menstrual pads. Laid end to end, these pads would stretch 1.6 million miles. That's enough for three round trips to the moon! Another 7 billion tampons go into landfills, sewers, and waterways every year. Besides creating a huge waste disposal problem, disposable pads and tampons waste natural resources. Making these products also pollutes the environment. The materials used in most menstrual pads in the United States release dioxin and other pollutants into the environment.

A small but growing number of women are using cloth pads. They feel it's a matter of personal responsibility for the environment. They also argue that cloth pads are a healthier choice for women. Some of the companies selling these pads make them of organic cotton.

Used pads are soaked in cold water and then washed by machine. Most companies that make these pads also sell airtight, waterproof carrying cases for used pads. When you're at school or away from home, you put used pads in the carrying case. When you get home, simply drop them in a soaking pail until you are ready to wash them.

Reusable pads come in a variety of styles and thicknesses. They are available in many health food stores and co-ops. You'll also find a list of companies that make these pads in the Resource Section at the back of this book. The list includes the companies' phone number and e-mail, Web, or regular addresses, so you can contact them to ask for prices and ordering information.

Tampons

Tampons are small, tightly rolled cylinders of cotton or other absorbent material that are inserted into the vagina to absorb the menstrual flow. At the bottom of the tampon is a string which hangs out of the vaginal opening. You remove the tampon by pulling gently on the string.

Answers to FAQs (Frequently Asked Questions)

Here are answers to the top ten tampon FAQs:

1. *Yes, a virgin can use tampons.* (A virgin is a person who has not had sexual intercourse.) The tampon is inserted through the opening in the hymen that allows the menstrual flow to leave the vagina. Using tampons gradually stretches the hymen. Girls who use tampons usually have larger hymen openings than girls who use only pads, but the tampon has no effect on virginity. Neither does the condition of your hymen (see pages 77–80). You remain a virgin until you have sexual intercourse.

2. *Yes, a girl can use tampons right from the start.* Today many girls use tampons from the time of their very first period on. You'll find some tips for first-time users on pages 180–182.

---

virgin (VUR-jin)

3. *No, you can't push a tampon in too far and it can't go up inside you or get lost inside your body.* First of all, the vagina has only two openings. One is the external opening (where you insert the tampon). The other is the internal opening, at the top of the vagina, which leads to the uterus. This internal opening is no bigger around than a match head, so there's no way a tampon can go beyond the vagina. Sometimes, however, the string at the bottom of the tampon gets pushed up so that it doesn't hang out of the vagina. Luckily, this problem is easy to solve. (See page 183.)

   It's also possible that you might accidentally insert a second tampon before removing the previous one. This can cause the first tampon to become stuck crosswise in the upper part of your vagina. At first, you might not even feel the stuck tampon. But as soon as you find out it's there, you should remove the stuck tampon. Usually, this isn't too difficult. (See page 183.)

4. *No, you can't feel a tampon if it's been inserted correctly.* Once the tampon is in place, you won't even know it's there. If you can feel it, it's not far enough in. Just push it further in with your finger, or take it out and insert another.

5. *A tampon can't fall out.* Once a tampon is inserted, the soft vaginal walls mold around it. Tight muscles just inside the vaginal opening prevent the tampon from falling out.

6. *Yes, a tampon can leak even though you have it in properly and change tampons often.* Menstrual blood can seep down folds in the vaginal walls and out the vaginal opening, bypassing the tampon completely. If this happens to

you, you might want to wear a panty-liner pad for extra protection.

7. *No, you don't have to remove your tampon when you go to the bathroom.* You have three separate openings down there—the urinary, vaginal, and the anal opening. A tampon in the vagina does not interfere with either urinating or having a bowel movement. You can hold the tampon's removal string to one side when you urinate. If it gets wet, you can dry it off with a tissue or toilet paper.

8. *No, a tampon should not be used for absorbing vaginal discharge.* Vaginal discharge helps keep the vagina clean. It also helps prevent infections. You don't want to dry up the vagina by absorbing all the secretions into a tampon.

9. *No, you needn't worry that you'll insert the tampon into the wrong opening.* It simply isn't possible to insert a tampon into the urinary opening. It's far too small. And although it's physically possible to insert a tampon into the anus, it's highly unlikely you'd accidentally do so. For one thing, as soon as you inserted the tip, you would realize from the sensation you were in the wrong place.

10. *Yes, tampon users are still at risk for developing the rare but serious disease known as TSS (toxic shock syndrome).* However, today the risk is very small. In 1997, there were only five reported cases of TSS that were related to menstruation. This is down from a high of 814 cases reported in 1980. Much of the credit for this dramatic reduction goes to women who make sure they use tampons safely. Be sure to read the material on TSS (pages 168–169) before you start using tampons.

Choosing the Right Absorbency

To lower the risk of TSS, choose a tampon with the lowest *absorbency* rating that will still be able to handle your flow. Most brands come in three or four different absorbency ratings. The more a tampon can absorb, the higher the rating. Tampons with higher ratings are usually thicker than those with lower ratings. Tampons made for teens are usually thinner. All tampons in the United States use the absorbency ratings listed below. The rating is printed on the outside of the tampon package.

- LIGHT: This is the lowest rating. These tampons absorb the least and are used for light flow. They're usually the smallest and thinnest tampons. This means they're the easiest to insert.

- REGULAR: These can absorb more than the lights. They are good for light to medium flow.

- SUPER: These are still more absorbent. They work for medium to heavy flow. They are usually quite a bit thicker than the lights or regulars. This makes them difficult to insert for many young women.

- SUPER PLUS: These are even more absorbent. They are good for very heavy flow.

- ULTRA: This is the highest rating. These tampons absorb the most. They are usually the thickest tampons.

If you have to change your tampon more than every few hours, switch to the next highest rating. If your tampon is dry or sticks when you pull it out, it's too absorbent. Use one with a lower rating. Many women use tampons with different ratings on

---

absorbency (ab-SOR-ben-see)

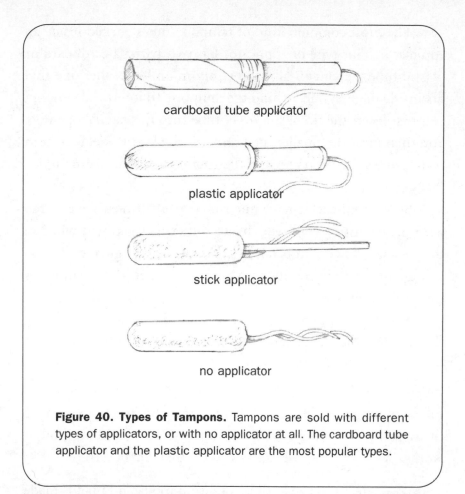

cardboard tube applicator

plastic applicator

stick applicator

no applicator

Figure 40. Types of Tampons. Tampons are sold with different types of applicators, or with no applicator at all. The cardboard tube applicator and the plastic applicator are the most popular types.

different days, depending on how heavy their flow is. But some girls can't insert the larger, more absorbent tampons comfortably.

Tampon Applicators

Aside from the absorbency, the main difference between different tampons is in the type of applicator used for insertion.

Some tampons don't have applicators. You use a fingertip to gently push the tampon into place. Other tampons come with a stick applicator. You guide the tampon into place with the stick. Then you remove the stick and throw it away.

The most common kind of tampon comes packed inside an applicator. This type of applicator has two parts: a cardboard or plastic tube which contains the tampon, and a smaller one that fits inside the first one, behind the tampon. To insert the tampon, you first insert the tip of the larger tube into the vaginal opening. You then push the smaller tube through the larger one, which, in turn, pushes the tampon out of the applicator and into the vagina. (See Figure 41.)

Some applicators have uncovered tips. Others are covered with little plastic petals, which can sometimes get bent while in the package. Since bent petals might scratch the vaginal walls, you should discard any tampons whose petals are not completely smooth and unbent.

Whatever tampon you use, read the instructions carefully. Wash your hands before and after insertion.

Tips for First-Time Users

Like anything new, inserting a tampon for the first time can be a little tricky. You might want to take one apart and see how it works. We've put together a few tips for first-time users.

- USE THE SLIMMEST SIZE: Light tampons and brands made especially for teens are the thinnest and easiest to insert.

- KNOW WHERE YOU'RE GOING: Get a mirror and look at your vaginal opening. Put a finger inside your vagina and tighten the muscles at the vaginal opening. These muscles keep the tampon from falling out. But you have to push the tampon far enough up into the vagina to get past these muscles. If you don't, the tampon will be trapped between the tight muscles. This won't injure anything, but it will be very uncomfortable.

- AIM IN THE RIGHT DIRECTION: Take a look at Figure 41. As you can see, your vagina doesn't go straight up and down.

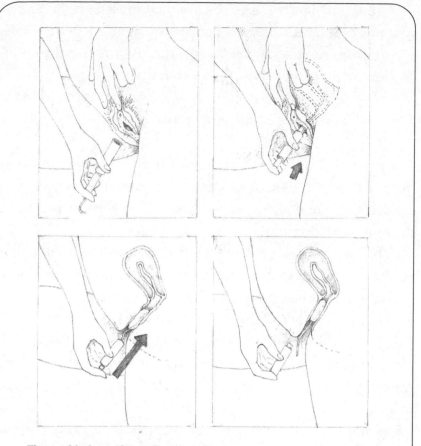

Figure 41. Inserting a Tampon. Tampons are small, tightly rolled cylinders of cotton or other absorbent material that absorb menstrual flow. They can be inserted into the vagina by means of a cardboard tube or plastic applicator.

Aiming the tampon straight up doesn't work. Instead, point it toward the lower part of your back.

- USE LUBRICATION: If your vagina is dry, use some K-Y Jelly. (K-Y Jelly easily washes off with soap and water. It's sold in most pharmacies or drugstores. You don't need a doctor's prescription to buy it.) A little lubrication on the tip of the tampon helps a lot. Don't use Vaseline or lotions, though.

- RELAX: If you're tense, your vaginal muscles tighten. This makes it hard to get the tampon in. Take a few slow, deep breaths, relaxing as you breathe out. As you breathe in and out, repeat to yourself, "This is not brain surgery. I can do this." Hundreds of millions of other women can, and so can you. It just takes a little getting used to.

If it's painful or you feel faint, stop. If the tampon won't go in, don't force it. The opening in the hymen is usually large enough for a tampon, but not always. (The hymen, remember, is the thin tissue that partly covers the vaginal opening.)

If your hymen opening is too tight to allow for tampon insertion, you can stretch it yourself. This should be done gently and slowly, over many days or weeks. As with tampon insertion, stop if it feels painful. Here's how you do it: First, put some K-Y Jelly on your finger. (Don't use petroleum jelly or any lotion that contains perfumes or chemical additives.) Insert your finger into your vaginal opening as far as is comfortable. Then apply pressure by pressing downward toward the anus. Keep the pressure on for a few minutes, then release it. You can repeat this several times during each session. The next time, increase the pressure. Slowly work your way up to inserting two fingers. Once you can do that, apply pressure to the sides of the vaginal entrance, too. Continue the sessions until you can comfortably insert a tampon.

Changing, Removing, and Disposing of Tampons

There are a few rules to keep in mind with tampons.

- CHANGE TAMPONS EVERY FOUR TO EIGHT HOURS: This reduces the risk of toxic shock syndrome. At night you should consider using a pad rather than a tampon. That way you won't need to worry about getting up to change the tampon to protect yourself from TSS.

- DON'T FLUSH THE APPLICATOR: It's okay to flush the tampon itself down the toilet (except with certain types of septic systems or really ancient plumbing). But don't flush the applicator or packaging (even if they say you can). They can clog the pipes.

- DON'T FORGET TO REMOVE THE TAMPON: Tampons are so comfortable, you may forget one, especially if your period is just about over. Leaving tampons in too long may increase the risk of TSS. If you've forgotten a tampon, don't panic. Just take it out as soon as you remember—which may happen when you notice an unpleasant odor. The odor should clear up on its own once the tampon is removed. If it doesn't, see your doctor.

- IF YOU CAN'T FIND THE STRING: Sometimes, the string works its way up into the vagina. Also, the tampon can get turned sideways in the upper vagina. If this happens, relax. The tampon can't get lost or go up inside you. Just reach up into your vagina and pull the tampon out. (This can be tricky if you have short fingers, but bearing down, as if you were making a bowel movement, should bring the tampon within reach.)

CRAMPS

Most of us have menstrual cramps at some time in our lives. Usually, the pain is only mild to moderate and does not keep us from our normal activities. But many girls have cramps bad enough to keep them home from school. About one in ten has severe cramps.

Cramps are felt in the lower abdomen. The pain may radiate to the lower back or down the thighs. There may be sharp, sudden pains, a constant dull ache, or just a feeling of pressure. The pain may come in waves. Some women complain of a feeling of heaviness in the vulva.

Cramps usually start with the menstrual flow. Sometimes, though, the pain starts a day or so before or after the flow begins. Cramps usually last for two to three days, but some women have them for only a few hours, while others have them during the whole period.

OVER-THE-COUNTER PAIN RELIEVERS

We know that prostaglandins play a role in causing menstrual cramps. So the best over-the-counter products for cramps are those that both block the action of prostaglandins and relieve pain. If you are under twelve years old, consult your parents or doctor before using any of these medications.

- IBUPROFEN (brand names Midol, Advil, and Motrin) helps block prostaglandins. It is often the best choice for menstrual cramps. In fact, before it became available over the counter, doctors often prescribed it for cramps. Manufacturers often sell different pain relievers under the same brand name. Carefully read the label on the product you've chosen. Be sure it really does have ibuprofen in it.

  To get the most benefit from ibuprofen, you have to take it correctly. Start taking it as soon as your period starts and keep taking it for the first two days. (If your periods are regular or you have body signals, like breast tenderness or bloating, you may know when your period is close. If so, start taking ibuprofen a day or so before your period starts.) Continue for the first two

There may be other symptoms along with the cramps. Some women have nausea, vomiting, constipation, or diarrhea. Some feel tired, have headaches, feel dizzy, or even faint.

What Causes Cramps?

Sometimes cramps are the result of an underlying disease or medical problem. But in most cases, there is no underlying disease to account for the cramps. In the past, when doctors couldn't find a cause for cramps they often assumed it was all in the woman's head.

---

days of your period. Never take more than the amount recommended on the label.

- NAPROXEN SODIUM (brand name Aleve) is the newest over-the-counter product for menstrual cramps. Like ibuprofen, naproxen sodium blocks prostaglandins. In fact, the two drugs appear to act similarly. Some women respond better to one or the other, just because of individual differences in body chemistry.

- ASPIRIN blocks prostaglandins. But women under twenty should not take aspirin for cramps. (There is a risk of Reye's syndrome, a rare but serious disease.)

- ACETAMINOPHEN, sold under brand names such as Tylenol or Datril, is another popular painkiller. However, acetaminophen does not block prostaglandins. For this reason, it's not a good choice for menstrual cramps.

---

ibuprofen (eye-byou-PROH-fuhn)
naproxen sodium (nuh-PRAHK-suhn SOH-dee-uhm)
aspirin (ASS-puh-ruhn)
acetaminophen (uh-see-tuh-MIH-noh-fuhn)

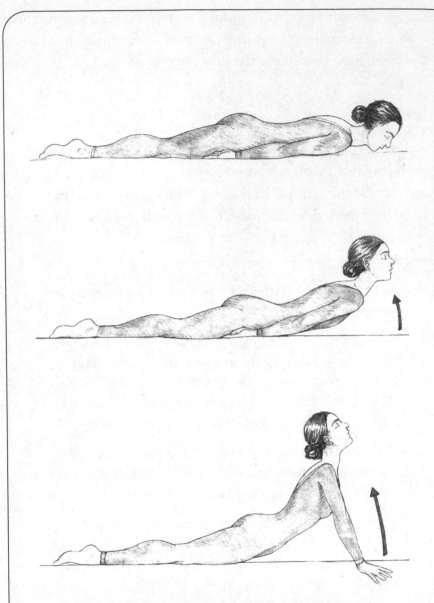

Exercise 1. Gradually raise your head and chest without using your arms until your torso is off the floor. Using your arms, further raise your torso so that your back is arched. Repeat several times.

Figure 42. Exercises for Menstrual Cramps

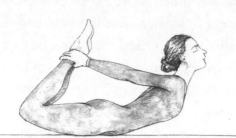

Exercise 2. Begin by lying on your stomach. Grab your ankles with both hands, pulling forward toward the back of your head. Gently rock back and forth. Repeat several times.

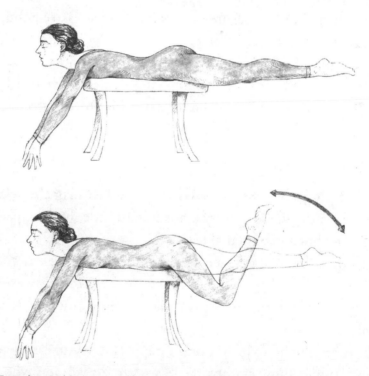

Exercise 3. Lie on a coffee table or platform as shown here. Place your hands on the floor in front of you. Bend your knees and pull your ankles in toward your buttocks. Then in one smooth continuous motion, kick your legs out again. Build up to doing it for six minutes.

Today we know much more about cramps. We now know the problem lies not in women's heads, but elsewhere in their bodies. We don't yet fully understand the cause. But we do know that when the lining of the uterus begins to break down, the body releases a chemical called a *prostaglandin*. It causes the muscles of the uterus to contract. This helps the uterus to shed its lining. But some women produce too much of this chemical. As a result, the uterus contracts too strongly, causing cramps.

Coping with Cramps: What You Can Do

Sometimes simple measures and home remedies are enough. If not, there are treatments you can buy "over the counter" (without a prescription). If none of these work, see your doctor. A doctor can prescribe other treatments for cramps. Alternative treatments, like *acupuncture* or Chinese herbs, have also proven effective.

Home Remedies

Heat improves blood flow and eases cramps. It may also relax the muscles in the uterus. So try a hot water bottle, heating pad, hot bath, or a hot cup of herbal tea.

For many women, masturbating to orgasm eases cramps. Afterward, blood flows more freely in the area. However, the uterus contracts during orgasm. For some women, this makes their cramps worse instead of better.

A healthy lifestyle may be an important key to easing period pain. Studies show cramps are less severe in women who don't smoke or drink and who exercise regularly. Aerobic exercise is

---

prostaglandin (prah-stuh-GLAN-din)
acupuncture (ACK-you-punk-chur)

especially good because it brings oxygen to the tissues. This calms down the action of prostaglandins. Running, walking briskly, swimming, jumping rope, or anything that gets you breathing hard is good, but don't overdo it.

Even if you're not feeling up to speed, try to stay active. If you feel weak, try something easy, like walking.

The best exercise for cramps may be yoga. Try the yoga-type exercises shown in Figure 42.

With the painkillers listed on pages 184–185, you should carefully follow the directions that come with the product. Pay attention to any warnings. For example, if you have stomach ulcers, you should avoid taking ibuprofen. If you're under twelve, you should see your doctor before taking any over-the-counter pain relievers.

In this chapter, we've tried to tell you everything (or at least almost everything) about having periods. In the next chapter, we'll get into something that you might find even more interesting: boys and puberty.

8.

BOYS AND PUBERTY

As we go through puberty, we usually get some information about what's happening to our own bodies. It comes from our parents, our teachers, and our friends. A lot of times, though, parents and teachers don't tell us about the opposite sex. (They may think that knowing about the opposite sex will make us want to rush out and have sex.) Other girls may not know any more about this subject than you do. However, that doesn't always stop them from spreading a lot of misinformation.

But not knowing what happens in the opposite sex can make puberty more confusing than it needs to be. That's why, in this chapter, we talk about puberty changes in boys' bodies. If you're like most girls, you are probably pretty curious about this. (In fact, we wouldn't be surprised if this is the first chapter you read.)

SIMILARITIES AND DIFFERENCES

As you can see in Figure 43, boys change quite a bit as they go through puberty. In many ways, puberty in boys is similar to

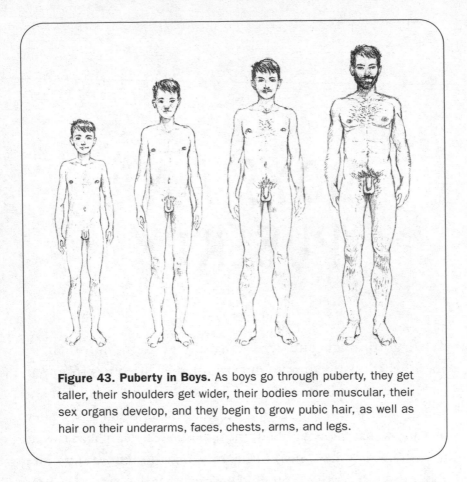

Figure 43. Puberty in Boys. As boys go through puberty, they get taller, their shoulders get wider, their bodies more muscular, their sex organs develop, and they begin to grow pubic hair, as well as hair on their underarms, faces, chests, arms, and legs.

puberty in girls. Both sexes undergo a growth spurt and develop more adult body shapes. Both boys and girls begin to grow pubic hair. The genital organs of both sexes develop. Boys start to make sperm for the first time, and girls produce their first ripe ovum. Boys and girls begin to perspire more and are likely to get pimples at this time in their lives.

But boys and girls are different. Some changes that happen to girls don't happen to boys. Obviously, boys don't menstruate. Also, there are changes that happen to boys that don't happen to girls. For instance, girls don't experience the same lowering and deepening of the voice that boys do.

The timing of puberty is also different in girls than it is in boys. Puberty usually starts later for boys. The average girl starts to develop breasts before the average boy shows any outward signs of puberty. She also begins to grow pubic hair before the average boy. Still, as we know, not everyone is average. Some boys start earlier than average. Boys who are early starters may enter puberty before some girls of the same age.

Even though boys and girls don't go through all the same changes, their feelings and emotional reactions to growing up are very similar.

THE FIRST CHANGES

For most boys, the first sign of puberty comes when their testicles and scrotum begin to develop. This change happens at a wide range of ages. A boy may start puberty when he's only nine. Or his testicles and scrotum may not start to develop until he's nearly fourteen or even older. On the average, boys start puberty when they're ten to twelve years old.

THE PENIS AND SCROTUM

Figure 2 on page 6 shows the sex organs on the outside of a man's body. You might want to take another look at that picture before reading on in this chapter. It will help you remember the names of the various parts of the male genitals.

The penis is made up of spongy tissue. On the inside is a hollow tube called the urethra, which runs the length of the penis. When a male *urinates*, the urine passes through this tube and comes out an opening at the tip of the glans. When a man ejacu-

---

urinates (YOUR-uh-nates)

lates, sperm also travel through this tube and come out of the same opening. Behind the penis lies the scrotum. It holds the two testicles. A boy's testicles are very sensitive and it can be very painful if they are hit or knocked about.

A boy's penis and scrotum change as he goes through puberty. During childhood, the skin of the scrotum is tight and the testicles are always drawn up close to the body. During puberty, the scrotum gets looser and the testicles usually hang down. Sometimes, though, when a boy is cold or frightened or having sexual feelings, his scrotum will tighten and draw the testicles up close to his body for a while.

Circumcision

The penis on the left side of Figure 44 has been circumcised. The foreskin has been removed. You can see all of the glans, or head, of the penis. Circumcision is usually done shortly after a boy is born, but not all males are circumcised. The penis shown on the right side of Figure 44 has not been circumcised. In this drawing the foreskin covers all of the glans. Some foreskins are longer than the one shown here. Others are shorter. Shorter ones cover less of the glans. Longer ones may extend beyond, or overhang, the glans.

The foreskin of an adult male's uncircumcised penis can be retracted, or pulled back down on the shaft of the penis. The foreskin is actually two layers thick. The two layers glide back and forth over each other. This gliding action allows the foreskin to be retracted. The inner layer isn't really skin at all. It is a special kind of very sensitive tissue.

Today about six out of every ten male babies born in the United States are circumcised. Some Jewish and Muslim parents have their boy babies circumcised for religious reasons. Other parents have their boys circumcised for what they think are important

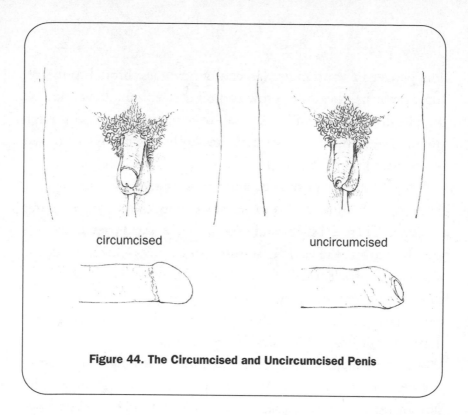

circumcised

uncircumcised

Figure 44. The Circumcised and Uncircumcised Penis

medical reasons. Still others have their babies circumcised because the father is circumcised.

It used to be thought that men who weren't circumcised were more likely to get infections or cancer of the penis. Today doctors doubt that being circumcised really reduces the chance that a man will get this type of cancer. Besides, cancer of the penis is very rare. And there is no real evidence that uncircumcised men are more likely to get infections. Uncircumcised babies are at a somewhat higher risk to get urinary tract infections, but these are usually easy to treat.

Nowadays, a lot of people question the medical value of putting a newborn baby through the pain of circumcision. More and more parents are deciding not to have their babies circumcised.

FIVE STAGES OF PUBERTY

The penis and scrotum get larger as a boy goes through puberty. Also, pubic hair begins to grow around the genitals. As you know, doctors divide breast and pubic hair development in girls into five stages. They also divide genital development in boys into five stages. (See Figure 45.)

Stage 1 starts at birth and continues until the boy starts Stage 2. The penis, scrotum, and testicles don't change very much during this stage. There is a slight and very slow increase in overall size.

In Stage 2, the testicles start to grow faster. They hang down more. One testicle usually hangs lower than the other. The skin of the scrotum darkens in color and gets rougher in texture. The penis itself doesn't get much larger during this stage. Most boys develop their first pubic hairs during this stage.

During Stage 3, the penis gets quite a bit longer and some-what wider. The testicles and scrotum continue to get larger. The skin of the penis and scrotum may continue to get darker. Boys who didn't develop it during Stage 2 will most likely get their first pubic hairs during this stage.

In Stage 4, the penis grows considerably longer and wider. The biggest change, though, is in the width of the penis. In addition, the glans is more developed. The testicles and scrotum continue grow-ing. The skin of the penis and scrotum may get still darker. A few boys don't develop pubic hair until they reach this stage.

Stage 5 is the adult stage. The penis has reached its full width and length, and the testicles and scrotum are fully developed. In this stage a boy has lots of curly pubic hairs. They grow on his lower belly and up toward his belly button. They may also grow down around his anus and out onto his thighs.

The age at which a girl starts puberty has nothing to do with how quickly she goes through its stages. The same is true for boys.

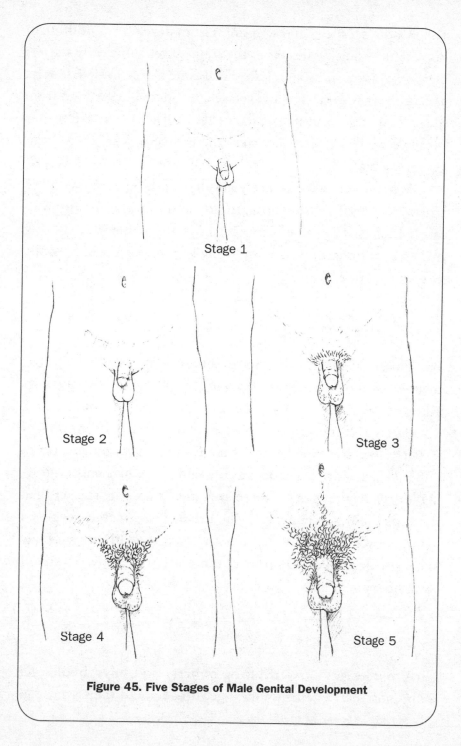

Figure 45. Five Stages of Male Genital Development

When a boy's testicles and scrotum start to develop has nothing to do with how quickly he gets to the adult stage. Some early starters develop quickly and some slowly. The same is true for late starters and for boys who start at an average age. Some boys will go from Stage 2 to Stage 5 in two years, or less. Other boys take five or more years. The typical boy takes three to four years to go from Stage 2 to Stage 5.

When a girl starts puberty also has nothing to do with the size of her breasts. Girls who start early don't always wind up with larger breasts. The same is true for boys and penis size. Starting early has nothing to do with how big a boy's penis will be when he's fully mature.

THE GROWTH SPURT

Like girls, boys go through a growth spurt during puberty. They start to grow taller and heavier at a rapid rate. Unlike girls, boys also have a strength spurt during which they grow stronger at a rapid rate.

For girls, the growth spurt happens at the beginning of puberty. For the average boy, the growth spurt comes later in puberty. Generally, it happens at the same time his penis is growing longer. At the age of ten or eleven, many boys are shorter than the girls their age. However, when their growth spurt begins a couple of years later, the boys catch up to the girls, and usually end up being taller. Of course, there are some boys who will always be shorter than a lot of girls.

CHANGING SHAPE

Girls' bodies get curvier during puberty and boys' bodies get more muscular. Their shoulders get broader and their arms and legs get thicker. This gives their bodies a less round and more manly shape. As with girls, boys' faces also change and become more adult. The change is often more dramatic in boys than it is in girls.

BODY HAIR, PERSPIRATION, PIMPLES, AND OTHER CHANGES

The hair on a boy's arms and legs gets darker and thicker during puberty. Some boys grow hair on their chests and sometimes on their backs, too. Some develop quite a bit of hair. Others have very little.

Like girls, boys develop underarm hair during puberty. (Boys usually don't shave this hair.) Perspiration and oil glands in the genital area, the underarms, the face, neck, shoulders, and back become more active in boys, just as they do in girls. Their body odor changes and they may start using deodorants or antiperspirants. Pimples and acne are likely to be a problem for boys, just as they are for some girls. On the whole, boys have more severe acne than girls.

Facial Hair

During puberty, boys also grow hair on their faces. The hair usually starts on the corners of the upper lips. Sideburns may start to grow at the same time. After the mustache fills out, hair grows on the upper part of the cheek and just below the middle of the lower lip. Finally, it grows on the chin. Hair usually starts growing on the chin after a boy's genitals are fully developed. For most boys, facial hair starts growing between the ages of fourteen and eighteen, but it may start earlier or later.

Breast Changes

Boys' breasts don't, of course, go through the same kind of changes as girls' breasts, but a boy's areola does get wider during puberty. Most boys' breasts swell a bit during puberty. Like girls, boys sometimes notice a feeling of tenderness or soreness in their breasts at this time. This swelling usually starts during Genital Stage 2 or 3. It may happen to both breasts or only to one. It may last only a few months or a year, or it may continue for two years or even longer. Eventually, though, it goes away.

Voice

Boys' voices change during puberty, getting lower and deeper. While their voices are changing, some boys' voices will "crack." That is, sometimes their voice will shift suddenly from a low pitch to a high, squeaky pitch. This cracking may last just a few months, but sometimes it goes on for a year or two.

ERECTIONS

Way back in Chapter 1, on page 13, we talked about erections. There are many slang terms for an erection. "Boner" and "hard-on" are just two of the terms used to refer to an erection.

When a boy has an erection, extra blood flows into his penis. It fills up the spongy tissue inside the penis. As the spongy tissue swells, it presses against blood vessels in the penis. This slows the flow of blood through the veins leading out of the penis. The spongy tissue then swells even more, making the penis hard. During an erection, the penis also gets longer and wider. It may also get darker in color. It stands erect, away from the body as in the drawings on the right side of Figure 46.

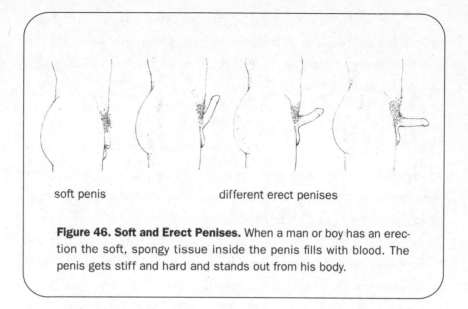

soft penis   different erect penises

Figure 46. Soft and Erect Penises. When a man or boy has an erection the soft, spongy tissue inside the penis fills with blood. The penis gets stiff and hard and stands out from his body.

Males get erections throughout their lives, even when they are tiny babies. Stroking or touching the penis can cause an erection. Getting sexually excited and having sexual fantasies can cause an erection. Males can also get erections even if they aren't feeling or thinking about anything sexual. Some males wake up in the morning with erections. Having to urinate can also cause erections.

Spontaneous Erections

During puberty, boys are apt to get erections more often than when they were younger. As they go through puberty, most boys start to have *spontaneous erections*. Spontaneous erections are erections that happen all by themselves, without any sexual feelings or thoughts.

A girl might be embarrassed by some of the changes that happen to her, like growing breasts, having periods, and so on. Similarly, spontaneous erections can be very embarrassing for a boy. They may happen when he is in school, at home, walking down the street, or just about anywhere. The boys in my classes have a lot of stories to tell about getting spontaneous erections. They all worry that people will notice the bulge in their pants caused by an erection.

Penis Size

Many girls worry about the size of their breasts. They may think their breasts aren't large enough. Boys have a similar kind of concern. Many boys think their penises are too small.

There's a lot of variation in the size of a soft penis, but size differences tend to disappear when the penis is erect. If a boy's penis is on the small side when soft, this doesn't mean it will be on the small side when erect. Also, boys sometimes forget that their penis doesn't reach full size until Stage 5.

Most adult men have erect penises between 5¼ and 6¾ inches in length. The average length is very close to 6 inches. There are a lot of myths about penis size. It simply isn't true that men with big penises are more masculine or better lovers. Penis size has very little to do with how much a woman enjoys sexual intercourse.

Getting Soft Again

When a male has an erection, one of two things may happen. The erection may go away all by itself. Or it may go away after he ejaculates. (During an ejaculation, muscles contract, causing a fluid, called semen, to spurt out of the penis.) In both cases, the penis gets smaller and softer as more blood flows through the veins leading out of the penis.

SPERM, INTERNAL SEX ORGANS, AND EJACULATION

Boys begin to make sperm during puberty. Figure 47 shows the inside of the testicle. Sperm are made inside the tiny thin tubes that coil up inside each testicle. Mature sperm look like tadpoles. But they are much smaller than the critter you see in Figure 47. They are too small to be seen by the naked eye. Once he's started making sperm, a male will usually continue making millions of fresh sperm every day for the rest of his life.

A boy's testicles do more than make sperm. They also make the male hormone *testosterone*. It's called the male hormone because it both helps to produce sperm and causes many of the

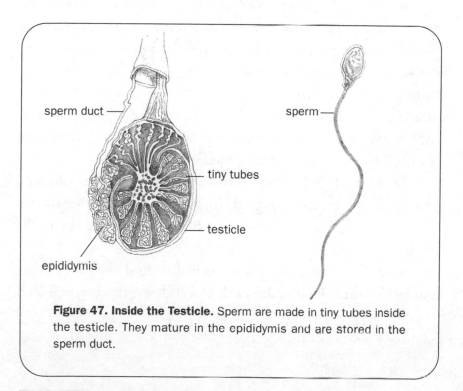

Figure 47. Inside the Testicle. Sperm are made in tiny tubes inside the testicle. They mature in the epididymis and are stored in the sperm duct.

testosterone (tes-TOS-tuh-roan)

changes boys go through during puberty. These changes include the growth of facial hair and muscle tissue, the broadening of the shoulders, and the lowering of the voice. And these are just some of the many changes testosterone causes.

The internal sex organs make and store sperm, prepare the sperm for ejaculation, and provide the route they take when they leave the body during ejaculation.

As we said, sperm are made inside each testicle. They then travel into the *epididymis*, which is a kind of holding tank sitting atop and behind each testicle. Sperm spend two to six weeks in the epididymis, where they finish maturing. The mature sperm then travel into one of two tubes, called *sperm ducts*, where they are stored.

In Chapter 1, you learned that sperm are released from the penis during ejaculation. At the beginning of an ejaculation, sperm are pumped to the upper ends of the sperm ducts and into the *ejaculatory ducts*. There they mix with other fluids that come from the *seminal vesicles* and the *prostate*. (See Figure 48.) This mixture is called semen. (The other fluids in semen nourish the sperm, providing energy for the long journey to fertilize an ovum.) The semen then enters the urethra.

In the final phase of ejaculation, powerful muscles contract and pump the semen through the urethra along the entire length of the penis. The semen comes out the opening at the tip of the penis in spurts.

Some girls are grossed out when they find out that semen and urine from the bladder both travel down the urethra. But

---

epididymis (eh-pih-DIH-duh-miss)
ejaculatory (ih-JACK-you-luh-TOR-ee)
seminal vesicles (SEM-in-uhl VES-uh-kuhls)
prostate (PRA-state)

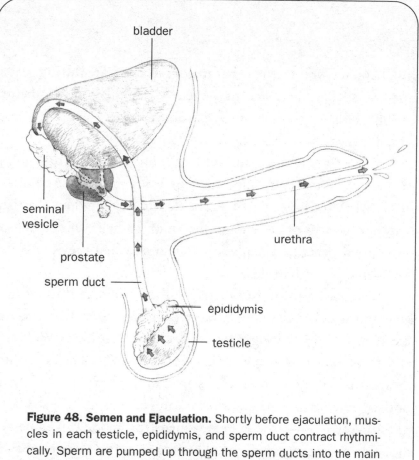

Figure 48. Semen and Ejaculation. Shortly before ejaculation, muscles in each testicle, epididymis, and sperm duct contract rhythmically. Sperm are pumped up through the sperm ducts into the main part of the body and into the prostate. Here the sperm mix with fluid from the seminal vesicles and prostate to form semen. At the time of ejaculation, more muscle contractions pump the semen through the urethra and out the urinary opening.

there's nothing gross or disgusting about it. Urine is just another liquid. Unless the male has an infection, his urine is germ-free. Besides, urine and semen don't travel through the urethra at the same time. A little valve closes off the man's bladder before he ejaculates.

FIRST EJACULATION, MASTURBATION, AND WET DREAMS

In Chapter 1, you learned that males can ejaculate during sexual intercourse. But most boys have their first ejaculation long before they begin having sex. As we'll explain, the first ejaculation may happen when a boy masturbates or during a wet dream.

Having his first ejaculation is a landmark for a boy going through puberty. It's as important for a boy as the first period is for a girl. Most boys ejaculate for the first time when they are between the ages of eleven and fifteen and a half. Of course, for some boys their first ejaculation will come when they are either younger or older than this.

Like most girls, most boys masturbate. They do this by rubbing and stroking the penis. Many boys have their first ejaculations while masturbating. Other boys have their first ejaculation in their sleep. This is known as having a *wet dream*. The boy wakes up and finds a teaspoon or so of semen on his belly or in his bedclothes. Having his first wet dream can come as quite a shock to an unprepared boy—the same way menstrual blood can come as a shock to an unprepared girl. This is just one example of why boys—just as much as girls—need information about puberty changes before these changes begin in their own bodies. Like girls, boys too want to know what is happening to their bodies.

9.
ROMANTIC AND SEXUAL FEELINGS

If a girl is thirteen and she's had her period and all she ever thinks about is boys and sex, is this normal?

—ANONYMOUS

Questions like this come up a lot because, as we go through puberty, many of us experience strong romantic and/or sexual feelings. For some girls, this means spending time imagining a passionate romance with a special someone or having sexual fantasies. For some girls, it means having the urge to masturbate more often. For some, it means getting interested in the opposite sex, having crushes, or having a romance.

These romantic and sexual feelings can be very strong. At times, it may even seem as if romance and sex are all you can think about. Some young people get so wrapped up that it's a bit scary for them. If you sometimes worry about how intense your romantic or sexual feelings are, it helps to know that these feelings are perfectly normal. A lot of people your age are going through the same thing.

Not everyone experiences such strong sexual or romantic feelings during puberty. Some girls are more involved in sports, school, music, or whatever. Sometimes we get questions like this:

How come all the other girls are totally into crushes and being in love and I'm just not?
—ANONYMOUS

Just as we each have our own timetable of development when it comes to the body changes of puberty, we also have our own timetable for romance and sexual interests. So there's no need to worry because everyone else your age is all wrapped up in romance and you're not. There's nothing wrong with you. Your personal timetable is just different from theirs. You have lots of time ahead of you to experience your sexual and romantic feelings.

The girls in my classes are curious about anything and everything having to do with sex. And they're especially curious about the kinds of romantic and sexual feelings that young people have when they're growing up. We talked about fantasies and masturbation earlier in this book. Having fantasies and masturbating are usually private things that you do by yourself. In this chapter, we'll be talking more about your sexual and romantic feelings that involve other people. We'll be talking about things like crushes, dating, and falling in love. But first, we'd like to say a couple of things about friendships.

JUST FRIENDS

When we're small children no one makes much of a fuss over the fact that two kids of the opposite sex are friends. Once in a while, people will make cracks about "puppy love." But it's just not a big deal if a little boy and girl play together, are best friends, or spend the night at each other's house. As puberty approaches, though, things change. Suddenly, it's no longer okay to spend the night at your best friend's house if your best friend happens to be someone of the opposite sex. The other kids at school or the adults around suddenly start assuming that you must be more than "just friends." They assume you like each other in a romantic, boyfriend/girlfriend sort of way.

At least, the kids in my classes often say that it's harder to be "just friends" after you reach a certain age. Here's what one girl in my class had to say:

> I'm going to Paul's Halloween party on Saturday, and my brother keeps teasing me, "Oh, you like Paul, you're in love with Paul." Well, I do like Paul, but not like that. All of a sudden, you can't just be friends with a boy. It's got to be boyfriend or girlfriend, like you're all romantic with each other.
>
> —ROSEMARY, AGE 13

An eleven-year-old boy had been friends with a girl since they were little kids. He had this to say:

> I went over to Hilary's house to spend the night, and we were swimming in the pool. These girls who live next door came over and they were saying things like, "Oh, you're playing with a girl. Oh, you're staying overnight at a girl's house. Oh, that's weird."
>
> —DONNY, AGE 11

Many kids complain about this sort of teasing and how people just assume that a friend of the opposite sex is more than "just a friend." So, in class, we talk about how to handle this problem. Here's some advice we've come up with:

- Just ignore the teasing and rumors. Take a "so what" attitude. After all, who cares if they think you're madly in love with your friend?

- Explain to people that you *are* "just friends." Tell them why you think it's fun or a good idea or whatever to be "just friends."

- Talk to your friend about it so the teasing or rumors don't make you feel uncomfortable around each other.

If you're having problems in this way, try some of this advice. Don't let the "romance thing" keep you from enjoying an opposite-sex friendship.

CRUSHES

Of course, sometimes we *are* interested in romance. In fact, many girls develop crushes. Having a crush means having romantic or sexual feelings toward a certain, special someone. Crushes can be very exciting. Just thinking about or catching a glimpse of the person you have a crush on can brighten your whole day. You may spend delightful hours imagining a romance with that special someone.

Sometimes girls develop crushes on someone who isn't very likely to return their affections. It might be a film star, a rock singer, a teacher, another adult, or a friend of an older brother or sister. These sorts of crushes can be a safe and healthy way of experimenting with romantic and sexual feelings. Still, no matter how much we may pretend otherwise, deep down we know that this person is unattainable, so we don't have to worry about real-life problems like what to say or how to act. We're free to imagine what we like, without worrying about whether that person will be attracted to us. In a way, having a crush on an unattainable someone is a way of rehearsing for the time when we will have a real-life romance.

But having this kind of crush can also be painful. One year some of the girls in my class developed crushes on a certain rock star. They plastered their bedroom walls with posters. They wore buttons with his face printed on them, pored over fan magazines, and had a great time sharing their feelings about him with one another. When the rock star got married, they were, naturally, disappointed, but one girl was more than disappointed. She was really upset. She had gotten too involved in her crush, and the rock star's marriage was devastating for her. If you find yourself developing a serious crush on someone unattainable, it helps to remind yourself from time to time that your crush isn't very realistic. This person isn't very likely to return your affections.

Not all crushes are unrealistic. You may develop a crush on someone near your own age whom you actually know through school, church, temple, or whatever. If that person shows an interest in you as well, the crush can be especially exciting. But yearning after a person who doesn't return your affections can hurt. If your crushes are causing you problems, it helps to discuss your feelings with someone. That person might be a friend, a parent, a teacher, another adult, or a counselor.

When girls talk with us about being romantically or sexually interested in someone they actually know, they often ask: *How do you find out if someone likes you? How do you let someone know how you feel?*

There are basically two ways: You can do it on your own, or you can have a friend do it for you. If you decide to have a friend do it, you'll want to pick someone you really trust. You don't want it known all over school. It's often easier to let someone else do the talking for you, but keep in mind that if you do this, you don't have very much control over what's being said. Suppose, for example, you only want your friend to bring up your name in a roundabout way and see how this other person reacts. Instead, your friend might make it sound as if you're madly in love with this person.

For these reasons, many people prefer to do it on their own. There are a lot of ways to let someone know how you feel. You can be friendly, start conversations, go out of your way to be around that person, ask the person to go out with you, or simply tell the person how you feel. You can also watch to see if that person does any of these sorts of things to *you*. If so, chances are that person likes you.

Regardless of whether you tell the person yourself or have a friend do it for you, make sure it's done in private. It may embarrass the person to talk about feelings for you in front of friends or classmates. As a result, the person might really like you, but not want to say so in front of everyone.

HOMOSEXUAL FEELINGS

Sometimes people have crushes on people of the same sex. When we talk about this in class it always brings up questions about *homosexuality*.

Homo means "same." Having *homosexual feelings* means having romantic or sexual feelings, fantasies, dreams, or crushes about someone of the same sex. Many boys and girls have homosexual thoughts or feelings or actual sexual experiences with someone of the same sex while they're growing up.

If you've had homosexual feelings or experiences, you may know that this is quite normal. You may not be at all worried

---

homosexual (ho-mo-SEK-shoo-uhl)
homosexuality (ho-mo-SEK-shoo-AL-eh-tee)

about it. Or you may feel somewhat confused or upset, or even downright scared, by these kinds of feelings or experiences. Perhaps you've heard people making jokes or using insulting slang terms when talking about homosexuality. If so, this may have caused you to wonder if your homosexual feelings or experiences are really okay. Perhaps you have heard someone say that homosexuality is morally wrong, sinful, abnormal, or a sign of mental sickness. If so, this, too, may have made you worry about your own feelings. If you've heard any of these things (or even if you haven't), we think it will be helpful for you to know the basic facts about homosexuality.

Almost everyone has homosexual thoughts, feelings, fantasies, or experiences at some time or another in their lives. That's why we usually consider people to be homosexuals only if, as adults, their strongest romantic and sexual attractions are toward someone of the same sex. Usually most of their actual sexual experiences will also involve someone of the same sex. About one in every ten adults in our society is a homosexual.

Both males and females can be homosexuals. "Gay" is a non-insulting slang term for either male or female homosexuals. Female homosexuals are also called *lesbians*. There have been homosexuals throughout history, including some very famous people. People from any social class, ethnic background, religious affiliation, or economic level may be homosexual. Doctors, nurses, lawyers, bus drivers, police officers, artists, business people, ministers, rabbis, priests, teachers, politicians, football players, married people, single people, parents—you name it—are homosexuals.

The majority of adults in our society are *heterosexual* people. *Hetero* means "different." Heterosexuals have strong romantic and

---

lesbians (LES bee-uhns)
heterosexual (HET-er-oh-SEK-shoo-uhl)

sexual attractions toward the opposite sex. Most of their actual sexual experiences involve the opposite sex.

We've talked about a few basic facts, but if you're like most of the girls in my classes you probably still have questions about homosexuality. Here are answers to a few of their questions.

Is homosexuality morally wrong? Is it unnatural, abnormal, or a sign of a mental sickness?

In the past, many people felt that homosexuality was sinful or abnormal. There are still some people who feel this way. However, nowadays, fewer and fewer people believe this. We feel that it's a personal matter, that some people happen to be homosexuals and that being homosexual is a perfectly healthy, normal, and acceptable way to be.

What's a bisexual?

A *bisexual* is a person who is equally attracted to males and females and whose sexual activities may involve either sex.

If a person has a lot of homosexual feelings or fools around with someone of the same sex while growing up, will this person be a homosexual as an adult?

Having homosexual feelings and experiences while you're growing up doesn't mean you'll be a homosexual as an adult. Many of the young people who have homosexual feelings and experiences while they're growing up turn out to be heterosexuals as adults. And quite naturally, some turn out to be homosexuals.

---

bisexual (bye-SEK-shoo-uhl)

We've talked to many adults who are homosexuals about their feelings when they were growing up, and have gotten many different answers. Some had homosexual feelings while they were growing up. Others had heterosexual feelings. Still others didn't have strong sexual feelings one way or the other as they were growing up.

Can people know for sure that they're gay even though they're still young?

Yes. At least some gay adults say that they knew they were homosexuals when they were teenagers. Some even say they knew when they were small children.

For more information about homosexuality, you can consult the Resource Section at the back of the book.

DATING

As young people move through puberty and into their teen years, many begin dating. This can be fun and exciting, but it can also create problems. For instance, you may want to date before your parents think you're old enough. Or you may not feel ready to date, and your parents or friends may be pushing you into it. You may have trouble deciding whether you want to go out with one person or go out with different people. If you've been dating one person regularly and decide you want to date others, it may be hard to end your steady dating relationship. Or if your "steady" wants to change the relationship, you may get hurt and have a hard time coping. On the other hand, you may want to date and no one is interested in going out with you. This could make you feel rather depressed.

Here again, if you're having dating problems, it might be helpful to talk them over with someone you respect and trust. You might talk to one of your parents, another adult you trust, a friend, or an older brother or sister. You might also want to take a look at our book *My Feelings, My Self*, which talks about these issues. In addition, it might be helpful for you to hear some of the questions that come up in my classes about this topic.

Suppose that you'd like to date, but you never have and you're beginning to wonder if you ever will?

If the other kids you know have already started dating, but you haven't, you may get to feeling that you won't ever start. If so, it helps to remember that we each have our own timetable when it comes to romantic matters, too. It can seem awfully hard if your personal timetable is moving along more slowly than other people's, but the fact that you're getting a slow start doesn't mean that you won't ever start dating. It may take a while, but eventually, you'll start dating, too. We guarantee it!

Remember, you've got many years ahead of you. It doesn't really matter if you start dating when you're only thirteen years old or not until you're twenty. What's important in the long run is that you feel good about yourself.

Is it all right for a girl to ask a boy out?

We think so. Although some people think it's not right or proper for girls to do the asking, most people don't see anything at all wrong with a girl taking the initiative. In fact, many people think it's a great idea. Almost every boy we've ever asked has said he wished more girls would do it. It's hard always having to be the asker! Girls are often in favor of this idea, too. However, many girls have admitted that they can't bring themselves to actually ask a boy out. They're worried about what others might think, or are afraid the boy might say "no."

We think girls should *go for it!* After all, whether you're a boy or a girl, the worst that can happen is that you'll be turned down. That wouldn't really be the end of the world, would it? One girl told us:

> My boyfriend is so shy. We'd never have gotten together if I hadn't gotten the ball rolling by asking him out. I'm glad I did!
>
> —CHANDRA, AGE 16

What if every time you ask someone out, the answer is "no"?

If you've asked a person out a number of times and the person keeps saying "no," you may just have to face the fact that this person doesn't want to go out with you. It can be difficult to know exactly how many times you should ask before giving up altogether. Partly, it will depend on what the person says. If you're told that the person is already dating someone else or simply isn't interested in you, that's pretty clear. You should stop asking. But if you're told, "I'm sorry, but I'm busy," you might want to try again. Perhaps the person would like to go out with you but really is busy. But if you keep trying and get this kind of reply each time, you might want to say something like, "I'd love to hear from you if you ever have some time free," and leave it at that. The person can then choose to follow up on that invitation or not.

If you've asked a number of different people out and all of them have said "no," you may begin feeling awfully discouraged.

You may even start to feel that something is so wrong or so horrible about you that no one will ever say "yes." But before you allow yourself to feel down and discouraged, think for a moment. Whom are you asking out? Maybe they're the wrong people! Are you asking only the best-looking or most popular people? If so, this may be part of your problem. For one thing, the best-looking and most popular people may already have lots of other people asking them out. Your chances might be better if you asked someone less popular or not totally gorgeous. Besides, the fact that someone is popular or good-looking doesn't necessarily mean you're going to have a great time on a date. What's more important is whether the person is nice. Can the two of you be comfortable with each other? Can you have fun together? A person's inner qualities are a lot more important than being popular or good-looking.

You might also ask yourself how well you know the person you're asking out. If you're asking someone you hardly know, this may be a big part of the reason you keep getting turned down. Take the time to get to know someone and let that person get to know you first. Then you're more likely to get a "yes" answer when you ask for a date.

It might also be helpful for you to have a mutual friend check things out before you ask for a date. Your friend can give you an idea of how the person might respond. If there's no interest, you'll save yourself the disappointment of being turned down. In addition, you might ask some of your friends who *they* think you should ask for a date. People love to play matchmaker. Your friends may come up with someone you wouldn't have thought of on your own. They may even know someone who's been dying to go out with you! So don't hesitate to ask for your friends' help.

Suppose you want to date, but your parents say "no"?

Young people usually choose to handle this problem in one of three ways: (1) Sneak around behind their parents' backs. (2) Go along with their parents' rules and wait until their parents say they're old enough. (3) Try and change their parents' minds. Let's look at each of these choices.

Sneaking around just isn't a good idea. If you get caught, you may get into a lot of trouble. Also, your parents may find it hard to trust you in the future. Even if you don't get caught, you'll probably feel awfully guilty about lying. And feeling guilty isn't much fun. In the end, sneaking around really isn't worth the price you have to pay.

On the other hand, it can be awfully hard to just go along with your parents' rules and wait until you're older. It's especially hard if there's a special someone you'd like to date. But parents usually aren't trying to be mean or unfair. They're trying to protect you from "getting in over your head" by dating at too young an age. Maybe they're right. If your parents say "no," ask yourself these questions: Are most of the other kids my age allowed to date? Would I really lose anything by waiting until I'm older?

If your honest answer to these two questions is "no," then perhaps waiting is the best choice for you. However, you may feel that your parents are being too strict or too old-fashioned. In that case, you might want to consider the third choice, changing their minds.

This may not be easy, but it's worth a try. For starters, find out exactly why they've made these rules. What are they worried about? Once you hear them out, you may be able to come up with a compromise. If, for instance, your parents think you're too young to go out on a solo date, maybe they'd allow you to go on group dates. Or if they won't allow dates for the movies, perhaps they'll allow you to go to a boy-girl party or invite someone to your house.

FALLING IN LOVE

Many young people fall in love, or at least what they think might be love, but how do you know when it's really love?

Emotions can't be weighed or measured. Different people have different ideas of what it means to be in love. So we can't tell you exactly what real love is, but we can share with you some of our thoughts on the subject.

We think it's important to recognize the differences between *infatuation* and true love. Infatuation is an intense, exciting (and sometimes confusing or scary) fireworks kind of feeling. You may be so wrapped up in your infatuation that it's hard to think about anything else. People sometimes mistake infatuation for love, especially because they may both start out the same way. But they're not the same. Infatuation usually doesn't last very long. True love does. In addition, you don't have to know someone very well in order to be infatuated, but in order to truly love someone, you have to know that person (both their good qualities and bad ones) very well. Infatuation can happen all of a sudden. True love takes more time. You may start out being infatuated and have it grow into true love. Or the infatuation may pass and you may discover that you aren't really "right" for each other after all.

Your relationship may start with the fireworks of an infatuation, or it may develop more slowly and gradually. In either case, a love relationship will sooner or later go through a questioning stage. One or both of you will question whether this relationship

---

infatuation (in-fat-chew-AY-shun)

is really a good one. During this questioning stage, one of you may decide to end the relationship. In our opinion, it's only after you go through this questioning stage and decide to stay together that you're really on the road to true love.

MAKING DECISIONS ABOUT HOW TO HANDLE YOUR ROMANTIC AND SEXUAL FEELINGS

Young people often face questions about how to handle their strong romantic and sexual feelings. When two people are attracted to each other, they quite naturally want to be physically close. Being physically close may mean something as simple as holding hands or kissing good night after a date. Or it may mean more than this. Physical closeness may even include something as intimate as sexual intercourse.

Some young people answer questions about how to handle their sexual and romantic feelings based on what they think everyone else is doing. Often they're wrong about what everyone else is doing. Besides, *just because everyone else does it does not mean it's right for you.*

Other young people just go along with what their parents or their religion says is right or wrong without really thinking much about it. Now, please don't misunderstand what we're saying here. We're not saying that you shouldn't follow your parents' or your religion's teachings or rules. In fact, we think parents and religions have excellent advice that's well worth following. But we've found that young people who accept, without question, what they've been taught sometimes run into problems. When they're actually in romantic situations, they often aren't able to stick to the rules they've been taught. The rules sort of fall apart in the face of tremendous pressure to experiment sexually. We think this sometimes happens because the rules weren't really theirs in the first place.

A lot of young people, maybe most of them, aren't at all sure what's right or wrong. They look for answers when it comes to deciding how far to go. If there were one set of answers that everyone agreed with, it would be easy. We could just tell you the answers. But it's not that simple. Different people have different ideas on these issues. So in class—especially in the classes for older boys and girls—we usually spend a good deal of time on this topic. We discuss making decisions about how to handle romantic and sexual feelings. We explain why people feel the way they do, without taking sides one way or the other.

Not until you give it some thought and decide for yourself what rules to follow will the rules become truly your own. And it's not until the rules are truly your own that they become rules you can live by.

When it comes to making decisions about sex, there are many things to consider. There isn't enough space here to cover everything you might need to know. For example, you can't make responsible decisions about sexual intercourse without being well informed about birth control and sexually transmitted diseases. (See the boxes on pages 226–227 and 228.) But before we leave this topic altogether, we'd like to answer a couple of the questions that often come up in our classes.

> *I'd like to have a girlfriend, but is someone my age (eleven) old enough to have sex?*
>
> *I'm twelve and there's a certain boy in my class that I like, and he likes me, too. I'm scared of having sex, though. What should I do?*

It's usually younger boys and girls who ask these sorts of questions. When I first heard questions like these, I was a bit shocked that boys and girls who were so young seemed to be asking questions about whether they were ready for sex.

However, in talking further with the young kids who asked these sorts of questions, I understood why they were asking these questions. It was because they often had very mistaken ideas about physical closeness. Some of them thought that kissing or being physically close in other ways happens as soon as you get involved with someone. Some thought that going on a date means you have to, at the very least, kiss the person good night or perhaps even go further. Some even thought that having a boyfriend or girlfriend automatically means that you're going to have sexual intercourse with that person.

These things just aren't true, but it's easy to see how kids get these mistaken ideas. In the books we read, it often seems as if two people who meet on one page are madly kissing each other on the next page. In the movies, it sometimes seems as if two perfect strangers take one look at each other, and the next thing we know they're in bed together.

Please don't be confused by what you read in books or see on TV or in the movies. Dating or having a boyfriend doesn't mean that you have to have sex or even kiss. Dating is, after all, a chance to get to know the person you're going out with. Once you know each other better, you may not want to have any kind of romantic or physical relationship. Above all, remember that when it comes to romance and sex, you're in charge. You don't have to do anything that doesn't feel right for you.

Is it all right to kiss on your first date?

Is it wrong to get into making out?

How far is "too far" to go?

Where should a person draw the line?

As we explained earlier, if everyone agreed on these issues, these would be easy questions to answer, but, of course, they don't. For instance, some people think it's not right to kiss on a first date, while others think it's perfectly okay to do so. Some people think making out is okay. Others don't. Some people think it's sinful to go beyond making out. Some don't think this is morally wrong, but are afraid that young people might get carried away and wind up going further than they really meant to.

Young people's answers to the sorts of questions listed above are strongly influenced by their personal situations. Their parents' values, their friends' opinions, their religion's teachings, their own moral beliefs, and their own emotional feelings are all important. These influences affect each of us differently, but we think the following guidelines can be helpful to anyone facing these questions:

- Whether it's tongue kissing, making out, or going further, don't let yourself be rushed into anything. Do only what you're really sure you want to do. After all, you have many years ahead of you; you can afford to wait until you are sure.

- Ask yourself how you feel about this other person. Is this someone you trust? Will this person start rumors or gossip about you? Are you doing these things because you really care about this person or simply because you're curious to try these things?

- Are you just trying to prove you're grown up, or trying to become more popular?

- Don't pressure someone into doing something he or she doesn't want to do. This pressure may take the form of a boy persuading a girl to go further than she really wants to. But boys are not the only ones to apply pressure. A girl may act like a boy isn't manly if he doesn't want to kiss or doesn't try to get her to go further.

- Don't allow yourself to fall for "lines" like these: "If you liked me, you'd make out with me." "If you truly cared about me, you wouldn't say no." "If you don't, I'll find someone else who will." "Everybody else is doing it." If someone hands you one of these lines, turn the line around. Tell the person: "If you truly cared about me, you wouldn't pressure me."

You may still be unsure about your own decisions and how to handle your sexual feelings. That's not surprising. There are so many aspects to consider—emotional, psychological, physical, spiritual, and moral (to mention just a few). It's always a good idea to wait until you're older, giving yourself time to consider all these things before you decide about sex.

In the end, of course, you're the one who decides. But you might find it useful to talk this over with other people. Don't (as many young people do) automatically rule out your parents as people to talk to. You may be surprised to find that your parents struggled with these same questions when they were your age. Often young people know that their parents' attitudes are more conservative or stricter than theirs. As a result, they may not talk about sexual decision-making with their parents. But even if this is so, your parents may have good reasons for feeling the way they do. And even if you don't totally agree with them, they might have things to say that could prove useful to you. You might also talk with an aunt or uncle, a sister or brother, or an older friend.

SEXUALITY: FEELING PRIVATE/FEELING GUILTY

Even though we haven't actually used the word *sexuality*, we've been talking about sexuality throughout this chapter. In fact, this

---

sexuality (SEK-shoo-ahl-eh-tee)

whole book is about sexuality. Some people think the word "sexuality" only applies to sexual intercourse, but it also includes things like your general attitudes about sex, feelings about your changing body, romantic and sexual fantasies, masturbation, childhood sex play, homosexual feelings, crushes, hugging, kissing, making out, and being physically close in other ways.

Feeling Private

Most people feel private, shy, or even a bit embarrassed about some aspect of their sexuality. Some young people, for instance, become

BIRTH CONTROL

If a male and a female want to have sexual intercourse, but don't want a pregnancy, they have to use some form of birth control. Some young people believe that you can't get pregnant the first time you have sex. This is *not true.* There are many, many women who have gotten pregnant the first time they had sex. Young people who have been having sex for a while without getting pregnant develop a false sense of confidence. They figure that since they've gotten away with it so far, they'll continue to get away with it. This is also *not true.* In fact, the longer a couple continues to have sexual intercourse without using birth control, the greater the chances of pregnancy. Some young people think, "It can't happen to me." They think pregnancy only happens to other people. Again, *not true.* Any couple having sex without using birth control may get pregnant, and most of them do sooner or later.

While we're on the subject of things that are not true, it is also not true that you can't get pregnant if you jump up and down after you have sex. This will not "shake the sperm out." It is not true that a female can't get pregnant if she has sex during her menstrual period. It is not true that douching after sex will prevent pregnancy. And it is not true very modest during puberty and no longer feel okay about family members seeing them nude. Some feel embarrassed asking questions or talking about the changes happening in their bodies. Some feel very private about starting their period or having wet dreams. They may not want their family or friends to know that these things have happened.

Private feelings can also center on romantic and sexual feelings or activities. Some kids are shy about the fact that they have a crush. Others feel embarrassed about their fantasies or about homosexual feelings. For most, masturbation is something that's very private. Young people may also feel shy about things like kiss-

that a woman can't get pregnant if a man pulls his penis out of her vagina before he ejaculates. During an erection, a male produces a few drops of fluid from the end of his penis. This fluid may contain sperm. Even if a man pulls out before ejaculating, he may still leave some sperm in the vagina. Also, if he ejaculates near the opening to the vagina, the sperm may still be able to swim up into the vagina.

Even if you're not having sex yet, it's a good idea to learn about birth control. There are many different methods. The *birth control pill* and the Norplant implant are two of the best methods of preventing pregnancy, but they require doctors' visits. Other methods can be purchased at the store without a doctor visit, but these methods may not be as effective as the pill.

Condoms are made of latex rubber and fit over the penis like a glove fits over a finger. They prevent the man's semen from getting into the vagina during ejaculation. The condom also helps to protect against sexually transmitted diseases. And you don't need a doctor's prescription to buy condoms.

There are many choices when it comes to birth control. It's important to become well informed so that you can eventually choose what is best for you. To learn more, see the Resource Section.

ing and making out, and other kinds of physical closeness. Some feel embarrassed even talking about these things, let alone actually doing them.

AIDS AND OTHER STDs

If you decide to have sexual intercourse, you also need to know about sexually transmitted diseases. Sexually transmitted diseases are also called *STDs, venereal diseases,* or *VD.* They are infections that are usually transmitted from one person to another through sexual contact. There are a number of different kinds of STDs. The most common ones are *gonorrhea, syphilis, chlamydia,* venereal warts, and *herpes.* Gonorrhea, chlamydia, and syphilis can be cured, but if they are not treated promptly, they can cause serious illness. There is no cure for herpes or venereal warts. Herpes has caused birth defects in the babies of some infected mothers. Venereal warts can increase the chance of getting certain types of cancer.

AIDS (acquired immune deficiency syndrome) is the most serious of all diseases that can be sexually transmitted. AIDS attacks the body's immune system and cannot be cured, but it is a manageable disease as long as you take your meds.

Because STDs are transmitted through sexual activity, people are often embarrassed to seek treatment or to tell their sex partners that they may have given them an STD. Before you have sex, you need to learn the signs and symptoms of STDs, how to avoid getting an STD, and what to do if you get one. To learn more about STDs, see the Resource Section, pages 244–245.

---

venereal (vuh-NEER-ee-uhl)
gonorrhea (gahn-uh-REE-uh)
syphilis (SIFF-uh-liss)
chlamydia (kluh-MID-ee-uh)
herpes (HUR-peez)

Some kids even worry about the fact that sexuality is such a private thing for them. But feeling private, shy, or even a bit embarrassed about sexuality is completely natural. It doesn't mean that you're hung up or uptight or that there's something wrong with you. It just means that you're normal!

Feeling Guilty

There is, however, a difference between feeling *private* about your sexuality and feeling *guilty* about it. Some kids don't just feel private, shy, or embarrassed. They also feel guilty, ashamed, dirty, or otherwise bad about some aspect of their sexuality.

When young people tell us they're having these guilty feelings, we suggest that they ask themselves this question: Is what I'm feeling guilty about something that is (or could be) harmful to myself or others? If it's not, then our advice is to try and let go of the guilty feelings. On the other hand, it may be something that is harmful. In that case, our advice is that you stop doing whatever it is that causes the guilty feelings. Also, make amends, if possible, and decide not to do it in the future.

Even when a person *has* done something harmful, it's often something that's not too serious. For instance, you might feel guilty because you've been flirting with your best friend's steady, but this isn't really all that serious. At least, it's not as serious as the kind of situation described by a fifteen-year-old boy. He felt guilty about having pressured his girlfriend to go further than she really wanted to:

> Making out is as far as she'd ever go because of her moral standards. I kept pushing and got her to, well . . . not actual intercourse, but further than she wanted to go. I didn't force her or anything. I was coming on strong, though. Now I feel like

some kind of pervert, and I can tell she doesn't feel good about herself. It's changed things between us. We're not so close.

—EDWARD, AGE 15

This boy did something that was harmful to his girlfriend's good feelings about herself and to his own good feelings about himself. It also hurt their relationship.

In other cases, the harm may be even more serious. For example, suppose a pregnancy resulted from rushing into unprotected sexual intercourse. In this case the harm done is quite serious indeed. Generally speaking, the more serious the harm, the harder it is to deal with the guilt. And even though you've changed your behavior and done what you can to make amends, this doesn't mean your guilt will go away completely.

It's important to remember that human beings are, after all, human. We do make mistakes. If you've done what you can to make amends and change your behavior, then try to forgive yourself and get on with your life.

We also want to remind you of the fact that different people have different ideas about what is or isn't harmful. Take, for example, masturbation, which is something many young people feel guilty about. Personally we think masturbating is a perfectly normal and healthy thing to do. Unless it goes against a person's moral principles, we usually advise young people who are feeling guilty about masturbating to try and relax and let go of the guilt. However, some people see things quite differently. They believe that masturbation is sinful or morally wrong and that people do themselves harm in a moral sense by masturbating. Because of these beliefs their advice would probably be just the opposite of ours. They might advise young people to stop masturbating.

How people react to situations where they feel guilty depends not only on how serious any harm done may be, but also on their ideas as to what is or isn't harmful. It's also possible for young people to feel guilty about doing something that few people would consider harmful at all. For instance, one sixteen-year-old girl wrote to us:

> If I just kiss a boy good night I feel so ashamed, not while I'm kissing but afterward. I know it's not normal to feel so guilty, yet I do. How can I get over feeling so guilty?
>
> —FRANCES, AGE 16

This girl felt guilty and ashamed simply for kissing a boy good night. And, judging from the letters we get, she's not alone. Some kids feel guilty even though they haven't actually *done* anything at all. For example, some girls have told us that they felt not just shy or embarrassed but also ashamed of the fact that they've gotten their periods.

Kids may feel ashamed or guilty about their sexuality even though they haven't done anything harmful. If so, they may find it helpful to think about *why* they feel this way. Often it's because some important person (often a parent) or group (maybe a religion) has taught them to feel this way. At one time many people in our society had *very* negative attitudes about sexuality. In your great-grandparents' day, sexual thoughts and feelings were often considered evil, the work of the devil. Sexual desires were considered impure or unclean, especially in women. Women who felt sexual urges or who enjoyed sex were considered abnormal, or perverted. Many people felt it was sinful even for married people to have sex, unless they were trying to have a child.

Of course, times change and so do people's attitudes. Today, most people in our society have more positive attitudes about sexuality. Still, many people continue to have negative, or at least somewhat negative, attitudes about sexuality. Parents who have these attitudes may pass them on to their children. Even though parents may not actually come out and say "Sexuality is bad," they may pass these attitudes on in other ways. A parent might, for instance, get upset when a little baby touches his or her sex organs and move the baby's hands away or even slap them. This may give the baby the idea that sex organs are nasty or dirty and that it's wrong or bad to touch them. When that baby grows up, he or she may feel ashamed about menstruation or wet dreams or may feel guilty about masturbating.

When you think about it this way, it's really not surprising that some kids feel unnecessary guilt about their sexuality. They feel guilty even though they haven't actually done anything that is harmful to themselves or others. It can be very difficult for these young people to let go of their guilty feelings. But being aware of where these feelings come from can help. People can and do learn to work past their guilt.

SEXUAL CRIMES

When we talk in class about making sexual decisions, I often find questions about sexual crimes in the "Everything You Ever Wanted to Know" question box. You too may have questions about these things.

Parents sometimes don't talk with their children about sexual crimes because they don't want to scare them. Many parents want to protect their children from even hearing about such terrible things. This is understandable, but the fact of the matter is, sexual crimes do happen. We feel that it's better for children to know about sexual crimes. Then they can be prepared to handle a situation where they might be victims of sexual crime.

Rape

Rape means forcing someone to have sex against his or her will. It can happen to anyone, to young children, to adults, to people of any age. Most rape victims are females, and most rapists are males. However, it's possible for a boy or man to be raped. Sometimes a male is raped by another male.

If you are a victim of rape, the most important thing is to get help right away. Some rape victims are so upset by what's happened that they just want to go home and try to forget the whole thing. But a rape victim needs medical attention as soon as possible. Even if the victim doesn't seem to have any serious injuries, there could be internal injuries that need medical attention. The victim also needs to be tested to make sure that he or she hasn't gotten a sexually transmitted disease. (These tests are one reason why a victim shouldn't bathe or shower before seeking medical attention.) If the victim is a female who is at least part of the way through puberty, she might want to take the morning-after pill to prevent pregnancy. (Girls have gotten pregnant even though they have not yet had their first period.) A rape victim also needs support to recover emotionally as well as physically, and should seek help for this reason, too.

If you are a rape victim, there are a number of ways to go about getting help. You can go to a hospital emergency room or call 911 and the police will take you to the hospital. There are rape hotlines in most big towns and cities. You can find the number of the hotline closest to your home in your telephone directory or by calling the information operator.

Child Sexual Abuse

Child sexual abuse may involve anything from touching, feeling, fondling, or kissing the sex organs to actual sexual intercourse. Incest is one type of sexual abuse. It involves one member of a family being sexual with another family member. Of course, it isn't incest when a husband and wife do these things with each other. Also, brothers and sisters often engage in some form of sex play as they're growing up. This may involve "playing doctor" or pretending to be "mommy and daddy." This kind of sex play between young children is very common. It isn't usually considered incest and isn't usually a harmful thing. But sexual contact between older siblings or with other family members is incest, and it can be very harmful.

Most victims of incest are girls who are victimized by their fathers, stepfathers, brothers, uncles, or some other male relative. It is also possible for a girl to be victimized by a female relative. Boys can also be victims of incest. When incest happens to a boy, it may be either a female or a male relative who victimizes him. Incest can happen to very young children, even to babies, as well as to older children and teenagers.

Incest isn't always a forceful thing, like rape. An older person in the family may be able to pressure the child into doing sexual things without actually having to use force. Most incest victims are so bewildered by what's going on that they simply don't know how to stop it or prevent it from happening again.

Child sexual abuse is considered incest only when the abuser is a family member. But sexual abuse can also occur when the abuser is a family friend, a teacher, coach, a parent's boyfriend or girlfriend, another adult the victim knows, or even a complete stranger. Boys as well as girls may be victims of this type of sexual abuse.

If you are a victim of sexual abuse, the most important thing to do is to tell someone. This can be a difficult thing to do, particularly if you are an incest victim.

The logical people to tell are your parents. (Of course, in cases of incest by a parent, you need to tell the other parent.) However, some parents have trouble believing their children at first. If, for whatever reason, your parents won't believe you, you might tell another relative, an aunt or uncle, a grandparent, an older sister or brother, who you feel will believe you. Or you could tell another adult, a teacher or counselor at school, a friend's mother or father, your minister or priest or rabbi, or any other adult you trust.

You can also call the Child Abuse Hotline. Their telephone number is listed in the Resource Section. The people who answer the phones are specially trained and they understand what you're going through. (Some of them have been victims of sexual crimes themselves.) You don't have to give your name, and what you say is entirely confidential, so don't hesitate to call.

Victims of incest and other types of childhood sexual abuse often find it hard to come forward and tell someone. Sometimes the person who committed the crime has made the victim promise to keep it a secret. But there are some promises and some secrets a person needn't keep, and this is definitely one of them. Or victims may find it hard to tell someone because they think that what happened is somehow their fault. They think they're to blame because they didn't stop it from happening, but this just isn't true. These crimes are always the fault of the older person. *The victim is never to blame and is never at fault in any way.* Some victims don't tell because they are afraid the person will harm them or get back at them for telling. But the police or other authorities will do whatever they can to protect the victim.

Incest victims sometimes hesitate to tell because telling could get the person who committed the crime into trouble with the police. Even though most victims hate what's been done to them, some of them still don't want to see a relative sent to jail. Although involving the police may seem like a horrifying idea, it will be better for everyone in the end. And it will protect any brothers or sisters who may also be suffering abuse. Besides, those who commit incest aren't always sent to jail. If possible the judge sends the person for some form of *psychiatric* treatment, while at the same time making sure that the victim is protected from further abuse.

Some incest victims don't tell because they're afraid that the family will break up. They fear that their parents will get divorced, or things will get worse than they are. But if incest is going on, things are already about as bad as they could be. The victim and the other family members also need help in dealing with the situation. However, no one can get the help they need unless the victim has the courage to take the first step and tell someone.

Most victims of incest and other types of sexual abuse feel a mixture of anger, embarrassment, and shame. This can also make it hard to come forward and tell someone. But you have the right to protect yourself from abuse. So even though you may feel embarrassed, it's important to tell someone. It's really the best thing for everyone.

If you have been abused, you may have concerns about what will happen when you grow up and choose to begin having sex. Many victims worry that future sex partners will be able to tell that they've been abused. But this is not the case. No one will know about the abuse unless you choose to tell that person.

Being abused does not physically impair your sexual ability, but abuse can have long-lasting emotional effects. If you've been abused, we strongly suggest you get counseling to help you recover emotionally. (You can call the abuse hotline number listed in the Resource Section for help in finding counseling in your area.)

A FEW FINAL WORDS

As you know, there are a number of physical changes that take place in our bodies during puberty. For most of us, these physical

---

psychiatric (sigh-kee-AT-trick)

changes are accompanied by certain emotional changes. For instance, we may feel very "up," proud, and excited by the fact that we're growing up and becoming adults. But along with these positive feelings, most of us also experience less-than-totally-wonderful feelings from time to time as we're going through puberty. It's not uncommon for young people to have the "blues," times when we feel depressed or down in the dumps, sometimes for no apparent reason. Part of the reason we have these feelings may be the new hormones our bodies are making. Hormones are powerful substances, and they can affect our emotions. It takes our bodies and emotions some time to adjust to these hormones, and some doctors feel that the emotional ups and downs many people experience are due, at least in part, to hormonal changes. But it's undoubtedly more than that. It's not just our bodies that are changing, it's our whole lives. At times, all this changing can seem a bit overwhelming, and we may feel uncertain, scared, anxious, or depressed.

One girl wrote to my daughter and me after she'd read the girls' book on puberty, expressing feelings that a lot of kids share. She said:

> I'm going through puberty right now and I'm very scared about it. Everyone says it's normal to feel this way, but every time I'm feeling good and everything, I suddenly get this depressed feeling and I don't want to grow up anymore. I just never want to get older and face things like possible rapes, diseases, deaths, etc.
>
> Also, I'm going to my first year of junior high school and I'm really scared. I'm not sure I'm ready to face all the changes.

It is quite normal to have these kinds of feelings. Knowing that other kids your age have the same feelings won't magically make you feel better, but it can help you to know that at least you're not alone.

Sometimes, young people are upset because they feel pressured to grow up all at once. As one boy put it:

Everyone I know is trying to grow up as fast as possible. What's the rush? I'm just not in a great big rush. I want to take my time. I'm tired of everyone trying to act all big and grown-up all the time.

And sometimes, the idea of being more grown-up and independent can be kind of scary. As one boy said:

Okay, so now all of a sudden I'm supposed to be all grown-up and have all these adult responsibilities. But I'm not ready to have these responsibilities and make all these decisions. In a few years, I'm going to go to college or maybe get a job and live on my own, and I don't even know what I want to do or if I can really do everything on my own. Sometimes I just want to stay a little kid.

However, there may be times when we feel that people around us, especially our parents, are keeping us from growing up as fast as we'd like to. One teenage girl expressed this point of view:

Sometimes I really hate my parents. They treat me like a little kid. They want to tell me what to wear or how I should wear my hair and where I can go and who I can go with and when I have to be home and blah, blah, blah. They're always bugging me. It's like they want me to stay "their little girl" forever and they won't let me grow up.

Going through puberty and becoming a teenager doesn't necessarily mean that you and your parents will have problems getting along with each other, but most teens do run into at least some conflicts with their parents. Indeed, at times it can seem like out-and-out war. These conflicts between teens and parents have to do with the change that takes place in the relationship between the parent and the child during these years. When we're little babies, we can't even feed ourselves, change our clothes, or go to the bathroom by ourselves. Our parents have to feed us, dress us, and change our diapers; we are *dependent* on them for everything. It's our parents' job to teach us how to take care of ourselves so that, eventually, we'll be able to go out and live on our own. And they have to take care of us and protect us until we're old enough to do that for ourselves. Children need their parents, but they also want to grow up, to be more independent, to take care of themselves, and to make decisions on their own. At the beginning of your teen years, you are still very dependent, but in a few years you'll be off to college or out earning your own living. So during your teen years, you and your parents are ending a relationship in which you're very dependent, and trying to establish a new relationship in which you are totally independent.

It's not easy to let go of old, familiar ways of relating and to establish new ones. Parents are used to being in charge, to making decisions. They may continue to tell you how to dress, how to wear your hair, what to do and when to do it, even after you feel that you're old enough to make these decisions on your own. This change in the relationship from dependent to independent doesn't usually come off without a hitch, and much of the stress, anger, and other negative feelings that you may experience during your teen years has to do with a working relationship with your parents.

Our relationships with our friends also change during these years, and here again, this changing can cause uncertain, confused, depressed, or otherwise difficult emotional feelings. Chances are you'll begin junior high and be going to a new school, making new friends, perhaps seeing less of old friends. Breaking old ties and making new ones isn't always an easy thing to do. During these years, being part of a certain gang or group usually becomes a very important part of your life. It can make things easier and more fun. But groups can present problems, too. You may find that you aren't accepted into a certain "in" group even though you'd very much like to be a part of it. Feelings of being "out of it" or being excluded from the group can make things seem very lonely.

Even if you are accepted by the group, you may find that there are still some problems. Being part of a group can have a lot of rewards—it helps us feel more accepted, more a part of things, less lonely and uncertain. But sometimes being part of a group "costs" us. We may have to act in certain ways or do certain things we don't feel good about in order to stay part of the group. Here's what some kids had to say about this:

> I really want to be "in" with this group of kids at school, but they do some things I don't like. Like they're always laughing at kids who aren't in the group, making jokes or comments and stuff when one of those kids gets up in front of class or something. I really want to be accepted, and it's not like I have to do what they do to be accepted. But if I do, I don't feel good about myself.
>
> —MARGIE, AGE 14

> I hate school 'cause I either have to act a certain way or be some outcast. Like in class, if you have an idea about something that is different than everyone else's, you can't say it or you'll be out of it and everyone will put you down. You have to do and say the same thing as everyone else or you're not okay.
>
> —TIM, AGE 13

Friends can talk me into doing things I don't really want to do. I'm in with the really "in" crowd, but the kids I run around with drink and sometimes smoke dope 'cause that's cool. My parents would kill me if they knew what I do, and really I'm not so into these things, but I do them to be part of the group.

—SHARON, AGE 15

Growing up is indeed a mixed bag of experiences. On the one hand, there are a lot of exciting things to look forward to; on the other hand, there are lots of changes—physical changes, life changes, changes in our relationships with our parents, our friends, and with the opposite sex. Probably at some time there must have been someone, somewhere, who went through puberty and the teenage years without a single problem, but we wouldn't bet a whole lot of money on it. If you're like most kids, you'll run into some problems as you go through the physical and emotional changes of puberty. We hope that this book will help in dealing with these problems. But this book is only a beginning; we've included a resource section at the end of this book that we think you'll find helpful.

RESOURCE SECTION

In this section you'll find books, websites, hotlines, and organizations you can contact for help or further information about topics covered in this book. The resources are organized alphabetically under the following headings:

- Birth Control, AIDS, and Sexually Transmitted Diseases (STDs)

- Counseling and Therapy

- Eating Disorders: Anorexia, Bulimia, Overeating, and Female Athletic Syndrome

- Gay and Lesbian Youth

- Menstrual Protection Products

- Resources for Parents and Teachers

- Sexual Harassment and Abuse

A NOTE ABOUT THE INTERNET

The sources in this section include Internet websites and e-mail addresses. All of us, and especially young people, need to be careful when we use the Internet. There are "adults-only" websites with lewd and offensive material. If you find yourself at such a website, leave that website. Many websites are really businesses that are trying to part you from your money. So *never give any business on the Internet a credit card number without first getting your parents' permission*. Also, don't fill out questionnaires that ask for personal information like your age, phone number, and address.

You can also talk directly to other people via Internet chatrooms and e-mail. Many people find this an entertaining way to correspond with other people. But this can be dangerous. Remember, people you meet and talk to on the Internet are complete strangers. They may not be anything like they say they are. Here are some commonsense rules for staying out of trouble.

- Never give your last name, address, Internet password, telephone number, or credit card number to someone you talk to on the Internet. Don't tell anyone what school you attend, where you go to church or temple, where you hang out, or any other information that could help someone find you. Immediately stop corresponding with anyone who asks for this kind of information.

- Never agree to meet someone you talk to on the Internet.

- Immediately stop corresponding with anyone who uses "nasty" language or in any other way makes you feel uncomfortable.

- If you're upset or puzzled by something that happens on the Internet, talk about it with a parent or some other adult you trust.

The Internet is a marvelous source of information. So follow the rules and be safe.

BIRTH CONTROL, AIDS, AND SEXUALLY TRANSMITTED DISEASES (STDs)

Books

Changing Bodies, Changing Lives: A Book for Teens on Sex and Relationships by Ruth Bell and others (Random House, 2005).

This is a great book for older teens. There are excellent chapters on birth control and sexually transmitted diseases. (Be sure you get the fourth edition, published in 2005, so you have the most up-to-date information.) The book also deals with a wide range of other issues, including sexuality, eating disorders, substance abuse, emotional health care, and safer sex.

Planned Parenthood (national office)

434 West 33rd Street
New York, NY 10001
Phone: 212-541-7800
Website: www.plannedparenthood.org
Hotline number: 800-230-7526

Planned Parenthood also has local chapters across the country. They provide birth control, pregnancy testing, testing and treatment for sexually transmitted diseases, abortion services or referrals, and other reproductive health information and services. You can call their 800 number for a clinic near you. Or look in the Yellow Pages under the headings family planning or birth control. Even if there's no Planned Parenthood clinic in your area, these headings should include listings for clinics that offer similar services to teens.

COUNSELING AND THERAPY

You don't have to deal with difficult emotional situations all by yourself. Difficult situations are a lot easier to deal with when you go outside yourself for help. There are many ways to find people who will listen to you and help you. You can talk to a parent or relative, to a friend, to a teacher, to a rabbi, minister, or priest.

There are also a number of ways to look for professional help in your area. Here are some:

- *Call a Hotline:* Look in the white pages under the headings: Teenline, Helpline, Talkline, Crisis Hotline, Crisis Intervention Services, and Suicide Prevention. If you can't find an appropriate hotline this way call a police station or a teen center and ask them for a hotline number. (You don't have to give them your name.) If you live in a small community with no hotlines then try the phone book of a large city in your area.

- *Contact a Teen Clinic:* Teen clinics often provide counseling services. Look in the yellow pages under Clinics. If you live in a small community with no teen clinics then try the phone book of a large city in your area.

- *Contact Your Church or Temple:* Ask your minister, priest, rabbi, or youth director to recommend a therapist or counselor.

- *Call a Radio Station:* Radio stations that broadcast mainly to teenagers or do talk shows for teenagers, may be able to recommend a counseling service. You don't have to talk on the air; just call them and say you need help.

- *Ask Your Family Doctor:* Your family doctor should be able to recommend a therapist in your area.

- *Contact a Mental Health Center:* Mental Health Centers usually offer teen services. Look in the Yellow Pages under Clinic or Health Services. Also look in the white pages under your county services.

- *Call the American Psychological Association:* This organization will give you a referral to a psychologist in your area. Their referral number is: 800-964-2000.

EATING DISORDERS: ANOREXIA, BULIMIA, OVEREATING, AND FEMALE ATHLETIC SYNDROME

National Eating Disorders Association

603 Stewart Street, Suite 803
Seattle, WA 98101
Phone: 800-931-2237
Website: www.nationaleatingdisorders.org
E-mail: info@nationaleatingdisorders.org

NEDA provides information and referrals for support groups and treatment of anorexia, bulimia, and binge eating disorders. For referrals to resources in your area call the number above, or visit the website and click on "Treatment Referrals." You can also request referrals via e-mail. Include your state, zip code, and the name of the nearest major city.

National Association of Anorexia Nervosa and Associated Disorders (ANAD)

P.O. Box 7
Highland Park, IL 60035
Hotline: 847-831-3438
E-mail: anad20@aol.com
Website: www.anad.org

ANAD is the oldest national nonprofit organization helping eating disorder victims and their families. It offers free counseling and information via hotline and e-mail. (Their hotline number, however, is not a toll-free number.)

In addition, ANAD offers free referrals to therapists and treatment programs across the United States and operates a network of support groups for sufferers and families. The organization publishes a quarterly newsletter and will mail customized information packets upon request.

Overeaters Anonymous (OA)

P.O. Box 44020
Rio Rancho, NM 87174
E-mail: info@oa.org
Website: www.oa.org

OA is a self-help group based on the same 12-step recovery program as Alcoholics Anonymous. There are no dues or fees to join or attend meetings. Their website contains information on OA and will help you find a meeting place near you. You can also e-mail them with any questions you have. Or call the nearest OA chapter for information and local meeting times. (Look in the white pages under Overeaters Anonymous.)

American College of Sports Medicine (ACSM)

Public Information Department
P.O. Box 1440
Indianapolis, IN 46206
Phone: 317-637-9200
Website: www.acsm.org

You can get a single copy of the ACSM brochure on Female Athletic Syndrome (or Female Athletic Triad, as it's often called) for free by writing to the above address. Include a self-addressed, business-size envelope that is stamped for two ounces of postage.

GAY AND LESBIAN YOUTH

Books

Young, Gay and Proud by Don Romesburg (Alyson Publications, fourth edition, 1995).

This is an excellent sourcebook for young people coming to terms with their sexuality.

Campaign to End Homophobia

P.O. Box 382401
Cambridge, MA 02238
Website: www.endhomophobia.org

This organization puts out two excellent pamphlets: "I Think I Might Be Gay . . . Now What Do I Do?" and "I Think I Might Be a Lesbian . . . Now What Do I Do?" You can write to the above address for a single copy of either pamphlet. (Include a self-addressed, business-size envelope that is stamped for two ounces of postage. Contributions to the Campaign, to defray the costs of developing and distributing this material, are always welcomed.)

National Gay/Lesbian/Bisexual Youth Hotline: 1-800-347-TEEN

This hotline for gay, lesbian, and bisexual youth is available 7 p.m. to 11:45 p.m. (Eastern Standard Time) Thursday through Sunday.

Parents, Families, and Friends of Lesbians and Gays (PFLAG)

1726 M Street NW, Suite 400
Washington, DC 20036
Phone: 202-467-8180
E-mail: info@pflag.org
Website: www.pflag.org

PFLAG is a national support organization with chapters throughout the country. Some of their excellent pamphlets are available at their website. Their pamphlet "Be Yourself" can also be ordered by mail. Send $2.00 for each pamphlet and request a free information packet and list of publications.

MENSTRUAL PROTECTION PRODUCTS

Several pad and tampon manufacturers have websites where you can see their products, and in some cases, order free samples. Alternative menstrual products such as reusable cotton pads and organic or non-chlorine-bleached tampons are sold in many health food stores. These products can also be purchased by phone or over the Internet and are listed below.

Tampon and Pad Manufacturers' Websites

Kimberly-Clark (Kotex pads, Lightdays Pantiliners, and Security tampons)
Website: www.kotex.com/na

Playtex (Sport, Beyond, and Gentle Glide tampons)
Website: www.playtexproductsinc.com/femcare

Johnson & Johnson (Stayfree pads,
Carefree Pantiliners, and o.b. tampons)
Websites: www.stayfree.com
　　　　www.carefreeliners.com
　　　　www.obtampons.com

Procter & Gamble (Tampax tampons and Always pads)
Websites: www.tampax.com
　　　　www.always.com

Alternative Menstrual Products

GladRags
P.O. Box 12648
Portland, OR 97212
Phone: 800-799-4523
E-mail: info@gladrags.com
Website: www.gladrags.com

This company sells reusable cotton pads and other alternative menstrual products.

Many Moons
Box 59
15-1594 Fairfield Rd.
Victoria, BC, Canada V8S 1G0
Phone: 800-916-4444
E-mail: manymoons@pacificcoast.net
Website: www.pacificcoast.net/~manymoons

This company sells reusable cotton pads.

Natracare
14901 E. Hampden Ave.
Suite 190
Aurora, CO 80014
Phone: 303-617-3476
Website: www.natracare.com

Natracare makes non-chlorine-bleached disposable pads and tampons.

Organic Essentials
822 Baldridge St.
O'Donnell, TX 79351
Phone: 800-765-6491
Website: www.organiccottonplus.com

This company sells tampons made of organically grown cotton and pads that are chlorine-free.

RESOURCES FOR PARENTS AND TEACHERS

Many of the resources listed under other headings in this section will also be helpful for parents and teachers. Under this heading, we've listed a few of our favorite resources for parents and teachers.

Books

From Diapers to Dating: A Parent's Guide to Raising Sexually Healthy Children by Debra W. Haffner (Newmarket Press, second edition, 2004).

This book is filled with sound, sensible advice and guidelines that will enable parents to deal wisely with a whole gamut of sexuality issues.

Hostile Hallways: The AAUW Survey on Sexual Harassment in America's Schools (AAUW, 1993).

This is the American Association of University Women's eye-opening survey on school sexual harassment.

How to Talk So Kids Will Listen and Listen So Kids Will Talk by Adele Faber and Elaine Mazlish (Perennial Currents, twentieth-anniversary edition, 2004).

Teaches basic communication skills that are invaluable for both parents and teachers.

The Kinsey Institute New Report on Sex by June Reinisch with Ruth Beasley (St. Martin's Press, 1994).

This comprehensive, basic reference contains information on a number of topics including puberty, anatomy and physiology, sexual health, and sexuality across the life cycle.

P.E.T.: Parent Effectiveness Training by Dr. Thomas Gordon (Three Rivers Press, revised edition, 2000).

This classic parenting guide teaches communication skills of value to parents and educators.

ETR Associates

4 Carbonero Way
Scotts Valley, CA 95066
Phone: 800-321-4407
Website: www.etr.org

ETR publishes and distributes materials on sexuality and health education for educators and parents, including books, curricula, brochures, videos, and other resources. You can browse their catalog online or write or call for a free catalog.

National Dissemination Center for Children and Youth With Disabilities (NICHCY)

P.O. Box 1492
Washington, DC 20013
Phone: 800-695-0285
E-mail: nichcy@aed.org
Website: www.nichcy.org

NICHCY is the national information and referral center that provides information on disabilities and disability-related issues for families and educators, including resources about teaching sexuality issues to children with disabilities. You can also get personal responses to specific questions via e-mail or phone.

Sexuality Information and Education Council of the United States (SIECUS)

130 W. 42nd Street, Suite 350
New York, NY 10036
Phone: 212-819-9770
Website: www.siecus.org

SIECUS is a national sex education advisory group. They have extensive materials for parents and teachers. Some of their excellent annotated bibliographies, fact sheets, and helpful brochures for parents are available online. You can also write or call for a catalog of their publications.

SEXUAL HARASSMENT AND ABUSE

Childhelp® National Child Abuse Hotline

800-422-4453 (800-4-A-CHILD)
800-222-4453 (800-2-A-CHILD; TTY for hearing impaired)
Website: www.childhelp.org

This twenty-four-hour hotline is set up to help young people and parents with any kind of abuse—sexual, emotional, or physical. You can talk to a trained person; just stay on the line! You don't have to give your name. The hotline also provides information and referrals regarding child abuse issues.

Equal Rights Advocates

1663 Mission Street, Suite 550
San Francisco, CA 94103
Phone: 415-621-0672
Fax: 415-621-6744
Hotline: 800-839-4ERA
Website: www.equalrights.org/publications/kyr/shschool.asp

This organization's website provides excellent information for young people and parents about school sexual harassment. They also have a free advice and counseling hotline. You can leave a message twenty-four hours a day and someone will return your call.

INDEX

(Page references in italics refer to illustrations.)

About the Authors

LYNDA MADARAS is the author of 12 books on health, child-care, and parenting, and recognized worldwide by librarians, teachers, parents, nurses, doctors—and the kids themselves—for her unique nonthreatening style, excellent organization, and thorough coverage of the experience of adolescence. For more than 25 years a sex and health education teacher for girls and boys in California, she conducts workshops for teachers, parents, and librarians, and has appeared on *Oprah,* CNN, PBS, and *Today.*

AREA MADARAS was just 11 years old when she assisted her mother with the first *What's Happening to My Body?* book. Now a communications consultant and mother of two, she lives in California and continues to assist her mother with the series.

The "What's Happening to My Body?" series by Lynda Madaras with Area Madaras

Available wherever books are sold or directly from the publisher.

The "What's Happening to My Body?" Book for Girls

$14.99 (paperback) 978-1-55704-764-9
$24.95 (hardcover) 978-1-55704-768-7

The "What's Happening to My Body?" Book for Boys

$14.99 (paperback) 978-1-55704-765-6
$24.95 (hardcover) 978-1-55704-769-4

My Body, My Self for Girls

$12.99 (paperback) 978-1-55704-766-3

My Body, My Self for Boys

$12.99 (paperback) 978-1-55704-767-0

Ready, Set, Grow! A "What's Happening to My Body?" Book for Younger Girls

$12.99 (paperback) 978-1-55704-565-2
$22.00 (hardcover) 978-1-55704-587-4

On Your Mark, Get Set, Grow! A "What's Happening to My Body?" Book for Younger Boys

$12.00 (paperback) 978-1-55704-781-6
$22.00 (hardcover) 978-1-55704-780-9

My Feelings, My Self (A Growing-Up Guide for Girls)

$12.95 (paperback) 978-1-55704-442-6

Parenting/Childcare Books